The Clean Eating Weeknight Plan

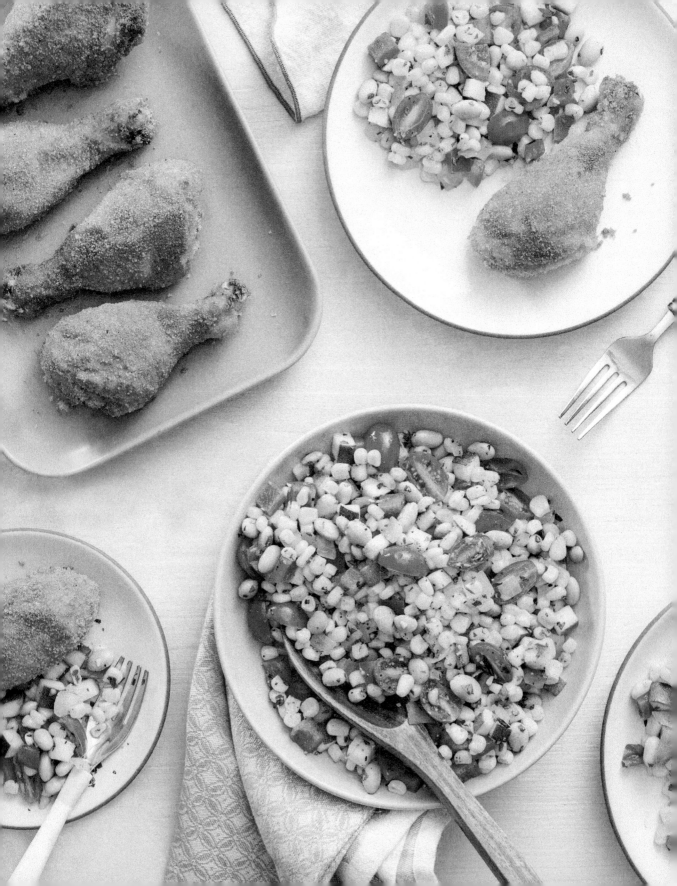

The Clean Eating Weeknight Plan

75 Clean & Simple Dinners Your Family Will Love

MICHELLE ANDERSON

ROCKRIDGE PRESS

I dedicate this book to my sons,
Mac and Cooper, who inspired me to come up with
healthy recipes to fuel all their adventures,
and to my husband, Scott, who tasted everything, even
the culinary experiments that weren't perfect.
Thank you for all your support and love.

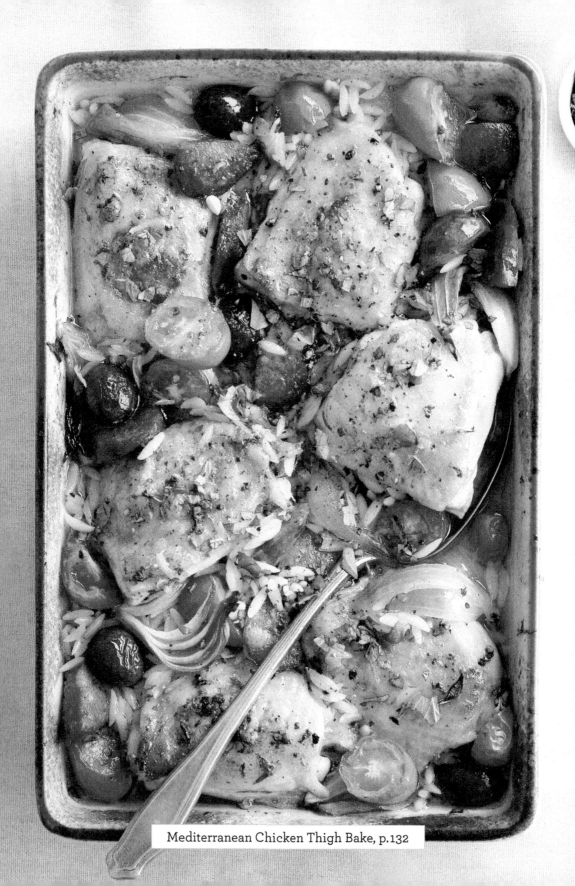

Mediterranean Chicken Thigh Bake, p.132

CONTENTS

INTRODUCTION

My fascination with food and good health started when I was young, thanks to the inspiration of my wonderful mother and her passion for living. My mother had the most incredible green thumb, so we enjoyed the bounty of our backyard garden throughout the summer months. Watching the glorious produce, still warm from the sun, blend with other whole-food ingredients in my mother's kitchen sparked my 25-year career as a professional chef. Although I experimented with almost every type of cuisine, I eventually found my personal and professional ingredient choices aligning with clean-eating concepts. My kitchen palette featured quality meats and seafood, nuts, creamy yogurt, olive oil, whole grains, legumes, and an abundance of fresh produce.

Clean-eating ingredients create delectable meals easily—with no fancy techniques required, and in very little time. This benefit was important to me as I worked insane hours in restaurants while still putting meals on the table for my growing family. Some nights I fell short of my nutrition goals for the kids (my husband feeding them saltine crackers and peanut butter for dinner comes to mind). Of course, thoughtful food choices are crucial for vibrant health, but sometimes lack of time and exhaustion from a long day make it difficult to follow through with good intentions. I was a professional chef with skills and time-saving techniques, and there were still days when creating a simple, healthy meal for my family seemed overwhelming!

That desire to prepare nutritious meals for my family and the challenge of handling multiple schedules inspired the creation of this book. These recipes follow clean-eating principles and can be created with just a few pieces of kitchen equipment and are quick to prepare. This makes clean eating the perfect lifestyle choice for busy families who value flavor and health.

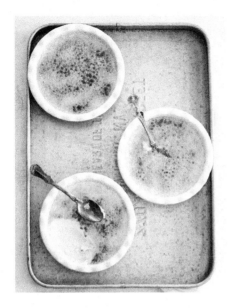
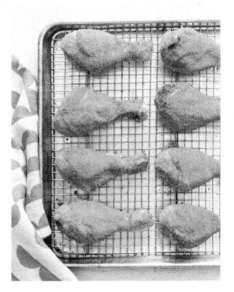

Some of the valuable tools you can take away from this book include:

- An understanding of clean eating and simple guidelines, such as foods to enjoy and foods to avoid.

- Tips to get the whole family eating clean.

- Strategies for clean eating when not at home, including how to navigate eating out.

- Suggestions for pantry staples and essential kitchen equipment.

- Three comprehensive midweek dinner meal plans, including shopping lists, make-ahead prep, and tips for leftovers.

- Ideas for clean-eating breakfasts and lunches.

- 100 clean-eating recipes to take the guesswork out of your meal planning.

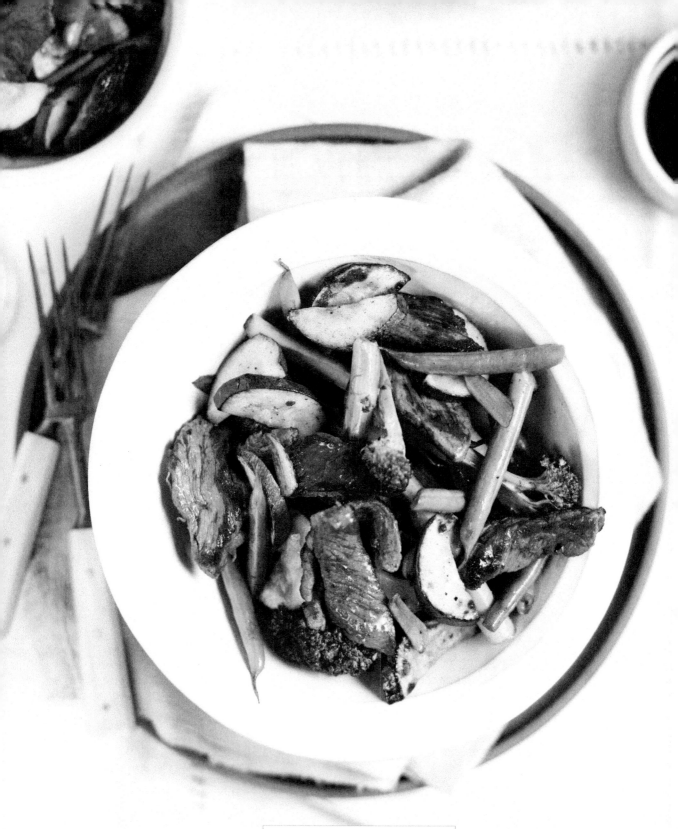

Beef-Broccoli Stir-Fry, p.148

1

WHAT'S FOR DINNER?

CLEANING UP YOUR ACT

You may already know all about clean eating and perhaps have been reaping the benefits for a while. However, if you're new to the concept, the guidelines are fairly straightforward: Clean eating involves choosing foods that are as close to their natural state as possible and excluding processed items, refined grains and sugars, and unhealthy fats. This is not a diet; it is a lifestyle change designed to promote good health, weight loss (if that is your goal), and lots of energy.

Food is certainly a delight, but it is meant to fuel your body instead of leaving you feeling hungry or deprived. Clean-eating meals are substantial and filling—you certainly won't be hungry! Best of all, clean eating is flexible and practical, so it can be sustainable in the long term. If you want to enjoy a slice of chocolate cake for your birthday, pick up your fork and dig in! If you decide you want to stick closely to clean-eating guidelines, you can also find delectable recipes for your favorite homemade desserts.

Because it's not a diet in the traditional sense, clean eating is not focused on what you can't eat, but rather on all the wonderful foods that you *can* enjoy. This balanced approach to eating includes all the food groups and features familiar ingredients. More a strategy than a diet, clean eating is meant to be flexible, so try to eat clean at least 80 percent of the time and don't stress if you indulge on occasion.

Here are the basic clean-eating principles for a healthier lifestyle:

Eat whole foods including vegetables, fruits, whole grains, legumes, and lean proteins. Eating foods as close to their natural state as possible and in a broad variety is key. Whole means unprocessed and unrefined so the foods are packed with nutrients and contain no harmful additives. You can include canned, packaged, and frozen foods that have whole-food ingredients, such as whole-grain pasta or sodium-free diced tomatoes. If you can afford them, organic or pasture-raised foods are wonderful additions.

Consume good fats and avoid bad fats. Your body needs healthy fats (monounsaturated fats, polyunsaturated fatty acids, and medium-chain saturated fats) to function properly. These fats serve as fuel, synthesize hormones, and are required for the absorption of fat-soluble vitamins. Healthy fats include olive oil, avocado oil, coconut oil, eggs, and fatty fish such as salmon. Unhealthy fats (trans fats and long-chain saturated fats) are found in many fried, processed, and packaged foods and can contribute to such health issues as obesity, diabetes, and cardiovascular disease.

Avoid refined sugar, refined grains, and processed foods. These foods are usually high in fat or calories (or both), high in sodium, and are empty of nutritional benefits. Removing them leaves room for foods that support vibrant health.

Combine lean protein, complex carbohydrates, and healthy fat in every meal. This helps stabilize blood sugar, releasing protein slowly into your bloodstream. The combination of these macronutrients can help you feel full longer and burn body fat faster.

Eat five to six small meals per day every two or three hours. This principle might be one of the hardest changes you make in your routine. Most people grow up eating three large meals a day—breakfast, lunch, and dinner—paying no attention to fluctuating blood sugar levels. Consuming small meals spaced throughout the day produces a continual influx of nutritious foods that help regulate blood sugar levels and provide consistent energy. Smaller meals mean smaller portion sizes, so be aware of the amount of food on your plate. For example, lean protein should be about ½ cup, carbs should be about ¾ cup, and vegetables and fruits should be about 1½ cups.

Always carry whole foods with you. Dinners might be the focus of this book, but clean eating happens all day. When you are at home, making a nutritious choice is simple, but it can be difficult on the go. Avoid the temptation of processed foods by packing your clean-eating meals and snacks in a cooler bag. (See breakfast or lunch suggestions in chapter 2, pages 21 and 29.)

Hydrate. Your body needs water to absorb water-soluble vitamins, to regulate body temperature, and to flush toxins out of your cells. Clean eating means always having filtered water on hand to sip all day, ideally half your body weight in ounces of water per day (e.g. if you weigh 140 pounds, drink 70 ounces of water).

FOODS TO ENJOY, FOODS TO AVOID

As with any eating plan, the list of foods you can eat and what you "have to" give up is of utmost interest, especially when you take your family into consideration. Remember, you will not be eliminating entire categories, except processed food, sugar, refined grains, and unhealthy fats. What's left is an abundance of choice! Basically, your meals will be delicious, colorful, and packed with nutrients. Every ingredient—from herbs to lean proteins—has a unique combination of macronutrients and micronutrients as well as antioxidants, so focus on variety. In no time, you'll automatically reach for clean-eating choices.

Use the following as more of a guideline than a comprehensive list of "allowed" foods:

Foods to Enjoy

- All fruits (fresh and frozen)
- All vegetables (fresh and frozen; sodium-free)
- Applesauce (unsweetened)
- Baking powder
- Baking soda
- Beef (fat trimmed)
- Canned tomatoes (sodium-free)
- Canned tuna and salmon (packed in water)
- Chicken (skinless, boneless)
- Cocoa powder
- Coffee
- Cottage cheese (in moderation)
- Cream cheese (in moderation)
- Dried fruit (in moderation)
- Edamame

- Eggs
- Feta cheese (low-sodium)
- Fish (except those that are high in mercury: tilefish, swordfish, shark, and king mackerel)
- Game meats (elk, venison, bison, buffalo, rabbit)
- Goat cheese (in moderation)
- Greek yogurt (plain)
- Green tea
- Ground beef (extra-lean)
- Ground chicken (lean)
- Ground lamb (lean)
- Ground pork (lean)
- Ground turkey (extra-lean)
- Hard cheeses (Parmesan, Asiago; in moderation)

- Herbal teas
- Herbs and spices
- Honey (in moderation)
- Hot sauce
- Hummus
- Kefir
- Lamb chops (trimmed)
- Lamb rack
- Legumes (black beans, black-eyed peas, chickpeas, kidney beans, lentils)
- Maple syrup (in moderation)
- Milk (fat-free)
- Mustard
- Nut butters (in moderation)
- Nut flours
- Nut milks
- Nutritional yeast
- Nuts (in moderation)
- Oils (avocado, coconut, sunflower, walnut; in moderation)
- Olive oil
- Olives
- Pickles
- Pork chops or roasts (fat trimmed)
- Pork tenderloin
- Protein powder (all-natural)

- Pure vanilla extract
- Salsa
- Sauerkraut
- Sea salt
- Seeds (chia, flax, pumpkin, sesame, sunflower)
- Shellfish (lobster, crab, scallops, clams, mussels, shrimp)
- Soba noodles
- Stevia
- Stock (vegetable, beef, chicken; low-sodium)
- Tahini
- Tamari (in moderation)
- Tempeh
- Tofu
- Turkey breast (skinless, boneless)
- Veal
- Vinegars (apple cider, rice, balsamic)
- Whole grains
- Whole-grain flours, breads, pitas, tortillas (whole-wheat, oat, quinoa, amaranth, spelt)
- Whole-grain pasta
- Whole-wheat bread crumbs
- Yogurt (plain, fat-free)

Foods to Avoid

- Alcohol
- Artificial sweeteners
- Foods high in saturated fats or trans fats
- Fruit drinks and cocktails (not labeled as juice or 100 percent juice)
- High-fat dairy (unless specified above)
- Hydrogenated oils
- Junk foods
- Preservatives
- Processed foods
- Processed meats
- Sugar
- White flour (and white-flour products)

A CHANGE IN YOUR MENU

Congratulations on making the switch to clean eating! This commitment produces many amazing health benefits and will change your relationship with food. Food is fuel for your body and you will appreciate the incredible range of tastes and textures in your clean-eating meals.

Along with all the positive changes, you might encounter some hurdles. As long as you are aware of them, you can overcome them and move on. Your pre-clean-eating life will determine this. For example, if you usually eat frozen meals for dinner, cooking everything from scratch could be challenging. Shopping could also be a shock because your cart will be filled with fresh produce, lean proteins, grains, and legumes. You'll need to spend some time reading labels on packaged items, looking out for ingredients you can't pronounce or don't recognize. But the extra time spent cooking and shopping is an investment in your health, and, after a while, clean eating will become second nature.

Why You'll Love It

Your reasons for wanting your family to adopt a clean-eating lifestyle are your own. These reasons could range from wanting better health, to having concerns about genetically modified foods. Along the way, you could discover other important benefits that will make you love clean eating even more:

The food is downright delicious and filling. Clean eating is one of the plans favored by bodybuilders because you actually get to eat lots of food and it tastes wonderful. The abundance of food in clean eating combines into meals and snacks that are easy to prepare and resemble many family favorites such as lasagna, burgers, and yummy casseroles.

Meals are easy to prepare. Clean eating doesn't involve complicated culinary techniques. You don't need to spend hours sourcing odd ingredients, as most of what you eat can be found at your grocery store or farmers' market. Another benefit of easy preparation is the opportunity to spend time with your family creating healthy meals together and talking about your day.

It's better for the environment. One clean-eating recommendation is to seek out seasonal produce. Because this produce does not travel thousands of miles to reach your table, you reduce your carbon footprint. Local, seasonal produce tastes better and packs more nutrition than items that sit in warehouses. Eliminating processed foods also means you aren't supporting a system that creates a burden on the environment through excessive use of resources to process and package foods.

You feel healthy. Clean eating produces tangible, positive health changes, the extent of which depends on the state of your health when switching to the plan. The steady influx of whole nutritious foods and elimination of sugar, refined grains, and processed items provides your body with all the resources needed for glowing good health. You might experience weight loss, a boost in energy, an improved immune system, better sleep, lower blood pressure and a better cholesterol profile, and healthier skin and hair.

You feel happy. This may seem like a bold statement, but the plethora of whole foods such as vegetables, fruit, fish, and legumes provides vitamins, minerals, and omega-3 fatty acids that can alleviate the physical effects of stress and may contribute to feelings of well-being. B vitamins and omega-3 fatty acids are linked to higher levels of the feel-good chemicals dopamine and serotonin, so eating foods high in these nutrients can create a happy mood and a calm mind-set.

Getting Everyone On Board

Clean eating might make perfect sense to you, but your family could be resistant to the transition. Keep in mind that change takes time. Don't get discouraged if everyone's not on board from day one. Eventually, your family will come around, especially if you employ the following strategies:

Explain your clean-eating decision. Be straightforward and highlight the health benefits of the new foods. Be enthusiastic and use age-appropriate explanations. After all, food should be fun and delicious, so make sure you get that across to your family.

Eat meals together. Life with my teenagers means they often want to eat in their rooms in front of computers, and my husband can be just as bad with certain sports on TV. This practice does not allow for mindful eating, which can help you focus on the textures and flavors of clean-eating meals. Whenever possible, make dinner a relaxing family event.

Resist the urge to nag. Don't guilt your family members if they hit the drive-thru or bakery. Instead, stay the course, serve delicious meals, and fill your house with healthy choices.

Ease them into it. Rather than spring potentially unusual ingredients on your family all at once, introduce them gradually and in familiar meals. For example, quinoa can be used in place of rice or as the base of a salad that is already a family favorite.

Take care with presentation. As a chef, I learned that people eat with their eyes first. Clean-eating ingredients are fresh and lovely; making it easier to serve well-presented meals that are a pleasure to eat (and seem to taste better!).

Make healthy snacks accessible. Every shopping day, I come home and fill a large container with cut-up vegetables. I place a container of clean-eating dip on top and leave the vegetables on the top shelf of my refrigerator. This is the first snack my family reaches for because it is handy—and delicious.

Include your family in meal planning. Being involved creates a feeling of ownership, and people tend to buy-in on activities they help plan. Let everyone choose a weeknight meal from this book or from other resources.

Allow treats. Many people (especially kids) will overindulge in cookies, chocolate, or salty snacks if they are forbidden to eat them. With a clean-eating mind-set, the occasional scoop of ice cream or handful of pita crisps is absolutely fine, because everything is done in moderation.

Don't buy unhealthy foods. If your cupboards do not contain sugary snacks, chips, or sodas then your family will not eat them. Removing temptation is often all it takes to help you stick to a new lifestyle plan.

Make clean eating fun. Food is one of the joys in life, so celebrate it! Visit farmers' markets, grow tomatoes on the patio, and create new recipes as a family. Name the new recipes after the person who created the dish, and you'll have a memory to cherish.

Those Picky Eaters

My kids have gone through various changes in food preferences over the years, including an entire year where one kid wouldn't eat eggs, mushrooms, or tomatoes. (He then suddenly decided he loved them one day.) Here are five strategies for dealing with the picky eaters in your family:

Hide unwelcome ingredients. Purée or finely chop produce such as carrots, sweet potatoes, zucchini, and dark leafy greens and add them to sauces, puddings, and snacks. This strategy is only a quick fix.

Serve familiar dishes. Recreate clean-eating versions of family favorites such as spaghetti and meatballs using whole-grain pasta, clean-eating marinara, and tasty turkey meatballs instead of processed or packaged items. Simply serve it and don't comment on any changes.

Avoid problem ingredients. Some picky eaters don't like certain flavors but are fine with most others. In this case, omit those ingredients from your meals. Most picky eaters grow out of food issues as their palate matures. If your picky eater is an adult, discuss the meal plan and adjust accordingly.

Set a good example. Try new recipes rather than staying in your culinary comfort zone. My kids are not allowed to say they don't like something if they've never tried it. There is a two-bite rule at my house. If they don't like it after trying it, they don't have to eat it.

Leave no choice. If your picky eaters are older, your best strategy is to serve your clean-eating meals and stock your kitchen with healthy choices. If the only choice is wholesome food, they'll eventually eat it. My 10-year-old held out for two and a half days before trying a stir-fry that had the dreaded mushrooms in it. He ate everything on his plate and asked for seconds.

Out in the World

It can be difficult venturing out in the world and sticking to a clean-eating plan, but if you are aware of the pitfalls, you can be ready with a defense. You'll want to steer clear of fast-food restaurants and coffee-shop chains. Small restaurants are often your best choice because they cook from scratch and many use fresh, locally sourced ingredients. There will be moments, such as during business get-togethers or parties, where clean-eating options are sparse, but don't panic. Choose items that look appropriate, then get back to clean eating when possible.

STICK WITH IT

One of the biggest challenges when eating clean is sticking to it when you are not at home with all your healthy food choices at your fingertips. Here are five tips to ensure your success:

1. **Prep.** One of my tasks every evening is to prepare veggies or fruit, nuts, dried fruit, and granola for the following day. I sometimes package an entire week's worth of items if they are nonperishable for grab-and-go snacks or lunches for the kids. If there are leftovers from dinner, separate them into different containers. You are more likely to tote your food if it is ready to go!

2. **BYOF (bring your own food).** Pack a cooler bag with a selection of your prepped meals and snacks.

3. **Research before eating out.** Most restaurants post their menus online so you can see what is available that suits your clean-eating plan. This makes it easy to decide where to eat near your work or when you are traveling.

4. **Ask questions.** Most servers are trained on the cooking techniques and ingredients of the dishes their restaurant offers. Find out what is made in-house and how menu items are cooked. Choose steamed vegetables or a salad instead of heavy side dishes, and ask for protein without fatty sauces.

5. **Be gracious.** When you are a guest in someone's home, never be preachy about your food choices, just eat items as close to whole as possible. If family members are aware of your plan, they may prepare appropriate dishes or have no issue with you bringing your own clean-eating foods.

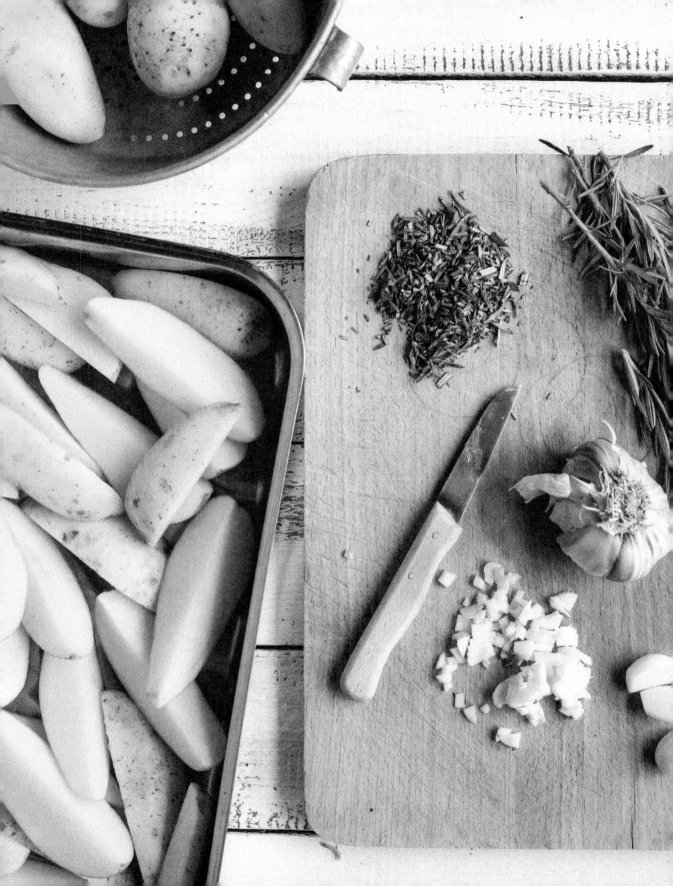

2

YOUR WEEKNIGHT MEAL PLAN

Maybe you're a veteran who creates comprehensive clean-eating meal plans and shopping lists with ease and you're just looking for new dinner recipes. If so, that's great! However, if you're new to clean eating or just want a hassle-free plan to feed your family during hectic weeknights, this chapter will serve as a valuable resource. On the pages that follow, you'll find three weeks of plans, each of which includes:

- Five dinner recipes
- Shopping lists
- A section showing what can be prepared in advance
- Suggestions for leftover ingredients or meals

The recipes selected for the three weeks are complete meals that do not require side dishes. If you wish to include sides, starters, or desserts, you'll want to revise your shopping lists accordingly. Also, if allergies or other dietary considerations need to be taken into account, substitute a recipe and adjust the shopping lists to meet your needs. All the recipes used in the meal plans include page numbers for easy reference; also, when perusing the recipe chapters, you will see a reference for the recipes in the meal plans.

KITCHEN PANTRY CHECKLIST

Having a well-stocked pantry makes life so much simpler, especially when you are following a clean-eating lifestyle. Having nutritious foods at your fingertips makes recipe creation a joy and reduces the risk of reaching for unhealthy snacks. The following list is not comprehensive, but does include the range of clean-eating ingredients found in the recipes that follow.

CANNED AND BOTTLED

- ☐ Broths (beef, chicken, vegetable; sodium-free)
- ☐ Legumes (black beans, lentils, garbanzo, navy, pinto, red kidney, white kidney; canned, sodium-free)
- ☐ Mustard (Dijon, grainy, hot)
- ☐ Red chili paste or hot sauce
- ☐ Tamari
- ☐ Tomato paste (sodium-free)
- ☐ Tomatoes (canned, sodium-free)
- ☐ Vinegars (balsamic, red wine, apple cider)

DRY GOODS

- ☐ Almond flour
- ☐ Baking powder
- ☐ Baking soda
- ☐ Brown rice
- ☐ Chia seeds
- ☐ Cocoa powder
- ☐ Coconut (unsweetened, shredded)
- ☐ Millet
- ☐ Nuts (almonds, hazelnuts, pistachios, cashews, pecans)
- ☐ Oats
- ☐ Quinoa
- ☐ Sesame seeds

- ☐ Whole-grain pasta (linguine, spaghetti, penne, farfalle)
- ☐ Whole-wheat flour
- ☐ Wild rice

FROZEN FOODS

- ☐ Edamame
- ☐ Peas

PANTRY ITEMS

- ☐ Coconut oil
- ☐ Curry powder and paste
- ☐ Herbs (oregano, thyme, basil, parsley, sage; dried)
- ☐ Honey
- ☐ Legumes (black beans, lentils, garbanzo, navy, pinto, red kidney, white kidney; dried)
- ☐ Maple syrup
- ☐ Molasses
- ☐ Nut butter (peanut, almond; natural)
- ☐ Olive oil (extra-virgin)
- ☐ Sea salt
- ☐ Sesame oil
- ☐ Spices (chili, cayenne, allspice, cinnamon, mustard, cumin, coriander, paprika, nutmeg, cloves, ginger, garlic powder, onion powder; ground)
- ☐ Vanilla extract (pure, organic)

ESSENTIAL TOOLS

You don't need any unusual or special tools to create the recipes in this book; they are designed to use as few pieces of kitchen equipment as possible. You probably already own some of the items listed under "Must Haves." However, there *are* some tools that could make your time in the kitchen shorter or more enjoyable. Here is a short list of essentials for your clean-eating adventure.

NICE TO HAVES

Slow cooker This appliance is used every week in my home, and several recipes in this book suggest the use of a slow cooker for convenience.

Barbecue The recipes in this book do not require a barbecue, but some can be grilled with lovely results, such as quesadillas, poultry, meats, and fish.

Immersion blender This useful handheld tool is perfect for puréeing soups or creating luscious sauces and smoothies.

Spiralizer This nifty tool creates long spiral noodles from vegetables and fruit for interesting salads and entrées.

Mandolin This manual cutting tool has several sets of blades (parallel and perpendicular) that cut produce into julienne, crinkle cuts, ribbons, and *bâtonnets* by sliding the ingredient down the deck.

Storage containers An assortment of sizes is convenient when you have leftovers. The recipes in this book are for the most part designed to serve four people so you will not need enormous containers. Look for 1-cup, 2-cup, and 4-cup sizes, as well as a few designed for dips or dressings.

MUST HAVES

High-quality kitchen knives This tool is absolutely essential. Well-honed, perfectly balanced kitchen knives save energy and time in the kitchen and reduce the risk of injury. At a minimum, select a quality chef's knife, utility knife, and paring knife.

Cutting boards Cutting boards are crucial for safe food preparation. If possible, get at least three, and designate them for meats/poultry, vegetables, and seafood.

Stainless steel bowls Nested bowls do not take up much room in your cupboard and can make prep work easy and quick. Stick to stainless steel because it does not discolor or rust.

Nonstick cookware At a minimum, purchase a large skillet, three sauce-pans (large, medium, and small), and a large stockpot for soups and stews.

Peeler and zester You can find both applications on one tool. Used for zesting citrus fruit, peeling ingredients, and creating nifty vegetable noodles.

Measuring cups and spoons The best recipe results often depend on accurate measurements. Make sure you have a complete set of wet and dry measuring cups and measuring spoons ranging from ⅛ teaspoon to 1 tablespoon.

Baking sheets Metal or silicone baking sheets with a 1-inch rim are very versatile for many recipes. If your kitchen has space, purchase half-size and full-size sheets.

Baking dishes You will use baking dishes for roasts, casseroles, stews, side dishes, and desserts. For the best results, buy an assortment that includes the following: 9-by-13-inch dish, 8-by-8-inch dish, and small 6- or 4-ounce ramekins.

Food processor or blender A food processor is best for puréeing soups or sauces (having a minimum 10-cup capacity), but a blender will create similar results. With a food processor, you can also grate vegetables.

WEEK 1
GETTING STARTED

If you are new to clean eating, Week 1 will be your opportunity to start this culinary adventure on the right foot! The theme of this week is getting familiar with your new clean-eating ingredients and shopping style. Depending on your current lifestyle, this might mean cooking from scratch every evening for the first time, or tweaking your meals to include delicious, wholesome ingredients. At the end of the week, you will start to appreciate the taste and texture of healthy ingredients prepared simply—and efficiently.

If you are just starting your clean-eating journey, don't stress about items in your pantry that do not adhere to the plan. Use items up where you can in recipes or donate them to a food bank or a relative. Then you can replenish your pantry, refrigerator, and freezer with wholesome clean-eating options.

DINNER MENU

MONDAY Mediterranean Chicken Thigh Bake *p. 132*

TUESDAY Primavera Frittata *p. 36*

WEDNESDAY Spicy Fish Stew *p. 117*

THURSDAY Basil-Lamb Burgers *p. 143*

FRIDAY Quinoa-Stuffed Acorn Squash *p. 94*

SHOPPING LIST

MEAT AND POULTRY

- ☐ Chicken thighs, boneless, 4 (5-ounce)
- ☐ Lamb, ground, 1 pound

SEAFOOD

- ☐ Fish (halibut, salmon, or haddock), boneless, skinless, 1 pound

DAIRY AND DAIRY SUBSTITUTES

- ☐ Almond milk, unsweetened, ¼ cup
- ☐ Eggs, 8
- ☐ Feta cheese, low-sodium, ¾ cup
- ☐ Goat cheese, ½ cup

PRODUCE AND HERBS

- ☐ Acorn squash, 2
- ☐ Basil, 1 bunch
- ☐ Carrots, 3
- ☐ Celery stalks, 3
- ☐ Cherry tomatoes, 1 pint
- ☐ Garlic, minced, 2 tablespoons
- ☐ Kale, 1 cup
- ☐ Lemon, 1
- ☐ Lettuce, iceberg, 1 head
- ☐ Red bell pepper, 1
- ☐ Red onion, 1
- ☐ Spinach, 2 cups
- ☐ Sweet onions, 4
- ☐ Sweet potato, 1
- ☐ Thyme, fresh, 1 bunch
- ☐ Tomato, 1
- ☐ Zucchini, 1

SPECIAL PANTRY ITEMS

- ☐ Basil pesto, ¼ cup
- ☐ Cranberries, dried, ½ cup
- ☐ Hamburger buns, whole-grain, 4
- ☐ Kalamata olives, ½ cup

REGULAR PANTRY ITEMS

- ☐ Brown rice, 1 cup
- ☐ Chicken broth, sodium-free, 3 cups
- ☐ Coriander, ground, ½ teaspoon
- ☐ Cumin, ground, ½ teaspoon
- ☐ Freshly ground black pepper
- ☐ Hazelnuts, chopped, ¼ cup
- ☐ Olive oil, 5½ tablespoons
- ☐ Quinoa, dried, 1 cup
- ☐ Red pepper flakes
- ☐ Sea salt
- ☐ Tomatoes, diced, sodium-free, 1 (28-ounce) can

Prep Ahead

- Cook the sweet potatoes for the Primavera Frittata.
- Make the pesto (if you are making it rather than buying it) for the Basil-Lamb Burgers.
- Make the patties for the Basil-Lamb Burgers.
- Cook the quinoa for the Quinoa-Stuffed Acorn Squash.
- Cook the acorn squash for the Quinoa-Stuffed Acorn Squash.

Leftovers

Several of the ingredients needed for the recipes will not be used up entirely. Here are some suggestions for leftover ingredients:

- Fresh basil from the Mediterranean Chicken Thigh Bake and the Spicy Fish Stew is also used for the homemade basil pesto for the Basil-Lamb Burgers.
- The remaining sweet onion (¾) from the Primavera Frittata is used in the Quinoa-Stuffed Acorn Squash.
- The remaining fennel bulb (¾) from the Spicy Fish Stew can be used in side dishes and salads.

CLEAN & EASY BREAKFAST IDEAS

Breakfast is often the most difficult meal to plan because mornings can feel rushed, and skipping this meal frees up time for other tasks. This is not ideal because breakfast is an important component in a healthy lifestyle. Breakfast is when you replenish the required calories and nutrients after sleeping all night: you *break* your night fast. Skipping breakfast almost guarantees you'll reach for sugary foods mid-morning or at lunch because your blood sugar is low. Clean-eating breakfast choices are diverse and can suit any type of schedule or dietary limitation.

Here are 10 breakfast suggestions to support your clean-eating lifestyle:

1. Leftovers from dinner or lunch the previous day; for example, any of the chapter 3 recipes: Quinoa-Stuffed Acorn Squash, Vegetable-Lentil Frittata, or Almond Rice Pudding.

2. Steel-cut or regular oatmeal, wheat berries, quinoa, or brown rice served with fresh fruit, chopped nuts, dried fruit, applesauce, or yogurt. Make in a slow cooker overnight or on the stove top in the morning.

3. Smoothies with nut milks, dark leafy greens, nut butters, fruit, vegetables, flaxseeds, maple syrup, and root vegetables.

4. Whole-grain pancakes, crêpes, or waffles served with fresh fruit, stewed fruit, root vegetables, nuts, seeds, nut butters, maple syrup, or a drizzle of honey.

5. Homemade protein cookies or bars made with whole grains, dark chocolate chips, dried fruit, nuts, seeds, maple syrup, and spices.

6. Eggs prepared in numerous, delicious ways such as poached, scrambled, sunny-side up, omelets, or soft-boiled and served with stewed tomatoes or beans, or wrapped in a tortilla or pita.

7. Yogurt or cottage cheese with cooked whole grains, granola, nuts, seeds, dried fruit, or fresh fruit.

8. Whole-grain muffins or quick breads served with nut butters and a bowl of fresh fruit salad.

9. Sweet or savory breakfast puddings, such as chia pudding with puréed pumpkin, root vegetable puddings, and custards made with nut milks topped with nuts, seeds, or fresh fruit.

10. Whole-grain toast topped with hardboiled eggs, avocado spread, nut butters, fresh fruit, or sliced tomatoes and goat cheese.

WEEK 2
KITCHEN EFFICIENCIES

Welcome to your second week of clean-eating weeknight dinners! This week is all about learning to handle your kitchen time efficiently and anticipating what might need restocking in your pantry. Reading the recipes for the weeknight meals should give you a good idea about timing and preparation. If one of your evenings is packed with activities or you have a late meeting, swap for another, shorter recipe for that day. The longest recipe this week is Hearty Vegetable Chili, which takes 45 minutes from start to finish.

If you are just transitioning to clean eating, you may be experiencing cravings for sugar or salty snacks this week. Satisfy your sweet tooth by making one of the delectable desserts in chapter 11, such as the Tempting Almond Butter Cups (page 165) or Chocolate-Zucchini Brownies (page 162). This will help curb any impulses to stray from your clean-eating plan. Don't worry, this lifestyle gets easier and becomes second nature before long!

DINNER MENU

MONDAY Beefy Stuffed Tomatoes *p. 146*

TUESDAY Shrimp with Roasted Peppers and Feta *p. 115*

WEDNESDAY Cottage Cheese Egg Bake *p. 40*

THURSDAY Turkey-Couscous Skillet *p. 127*

FRIDAY Hearty Vegetable Chili *p. 109*

SHOPPING LIST

MEAT AND POULTRY

- ☐ Beef, ground, extra-lean, 1 pound
- ☐ Turkey, cooked, 2 cups

SEAFOOD

- ☐ Shrimp, medium, peeled and deveined, 24

DAIRY AND DAIRY SUBSTITUTES

- ☐ Cottage cheese, 1 cup
- ☐ Eggs, 8
- ☐ Feta cheese, low-sodium, ½ cup
- ☐ Goat cheese, ¼ cup

PRODUCE AND HERBS

- ☐ Basil, 1 bunch
- ☐ Carrots, 1
- ☐ Cauliflower, 1 head
- ☐ Celery stalks, 2
- ☐ Cherry tomatoes, 1 pint
- ☐ Garlic, minced, 3 tablespoons
- ☐ Green beans, 1 cup
- ☐ Green bell pepper, 1
- ☐ Jalapeño pepper, 1
- ☐ Lemon, 1
- ☐ Parsley, 1 bunch
- ☐ Parsnip, 1
- ☐ Red bell peppers, 2
- ☐ Scallion, 1
- ☐ Spinach, 1 cup
- ☐ Sweet onions, 3
- ☐ Thyme, 1 bunch
- ☐ Tomatoes, 8
- ☐ Zucchini, 1

SPECIAL PANTRY ITEMS

- ☐ Israeli couscous, 1 cup
- ☐ Red bell peppers, roasted, ½ cup
- ☐ Wheat berries, 1 cup

REGULAR PANTRY ITEMS

- ☐ Cayenne pepper powder
- ☐ Chili powder, 3 tablespoons
- ☐ Cumin, ground, 1 tablespoon
- ☐ Freshly ground black pepper
- ☐ Navy beans, sodium-free, 1 (15-ounce) can
- ☐ Olive oil, 3 tablespoons
- ☐ Red kidney beans, sodium-free, 1 (15-ounce) can
- ☐ Red pepper flakes, ¼ teaspoon
- ☐ Sea salt
- ☐ Spaghetti, whole-grain, 8 ounces dried
- ☐ Tomatoes, diced, sodium-free, 2 (28-ounce) cans

Prep Ahead

- Cook the beef for the Beefy Stuffed Tomatoes.
- Cook the wheat berries for the Beefy Stuffed Tomatoes.
- Assemble the entire Cottage Cheese Egg Bake.
- Cook the turkey for the Turkey-Couscous Skillet.
- Cook the couscous for the Turkey-Couscous Skillet.
- Peel and devein the shrimp (if you buy them uncleaned) for Shrimp with Roasted Peppers and Feta.
- Roast the red pepper (if you are doing it from scratch) for the Shrimp with Roasted Peppers and Feta.
- Prep the entire Hearty Vegetable Chili recipe and set it up in a slow cooker.

Leftovers

Several of the ingredients needed for the recipes will not be used up entirely. Here are some suggestions for leftover ingredients:

- The parsley from the Beefy Stuffed Tomatoes can be used to accent any of the other recipes.
- The remaining cauliflower (¾ head) from the Turkey-Couscous Skillet is perfect for side dishes, salads, or as a snack.
- Leftover Hearty Vegetable Chili is fabulous over brown rice or spooned into a whole-wheat pita for lunch.

CUTTING COSTS
WHEN EATING CLEAN

Clean eating is not the most expensive lifestyle, but it certainly requires a larger budget than eating processed convenience foods. When you eat clean, your grocery cart will be filled with quality meats, poultry, seafood, and produce rather than cheap boxed meals or snacks. If you want to minimize the extra expense, here are some strategies you can adopt:

- Shop at farmers' markets and buy seasonally whenever possible.

- Create leftovers whenever possible so you can freeze the extra for another meal or enjoy a hearty lunch the following day.

- Serve vegetarian meals at least once or twice a week because these do not include pricey animal proteins.

- Make a weekly meal plan and a shopping list: Think about how many impulse buys you make when walking down the aisles at the grocery store. Having a comprehensive list can also eliminate multiple trips to the store for forgotten items.

- Buy items you use frequently in bulk, such as oats, brown rice, olive oil, nuts, and dried fruit.

LOW-FAT DAIRY VS. FULL-FAT DAIRY

The original clean-eating diet recommends only using low-fat or fat-free dairy in your meals because the fat in dairy is about 60 percent saturated fat. Since 2010, studies such as one published in *The American Journal of Clinical Nutrition* show that there is no evidence that saturated fat is linked to cardiovascular disease or stroke. On the contrary, saturated fat is essential for the absorption of fat-soluble vitamins such as vitamin A, D, E, and K. Saturated fat also acts as the building block for cell membranes and hormones in the body. Full-fat dairy products can make you feel full longer and actually contribute to a weight-loss-oriented or healthy diet.

WEEK 3
CREATING HEALTHY HABITS

Congratulations on starting your third week of clean eating! Two weeks without refined grains and sugar, unhealthy fats, and processed foods should mean you're feeling good. You may notice deeper sleep, more energy, and improved mental clarity during the day. The effects of all the nutritious food on your plate will be apparent. At the end of this week, your healthy food choices should become a set routine. As with the other weeks, take a look at the recommended recipes and see if there are changes you need to make, either with the timing or the recipe itself. Remember: Clean eating is a very flexible lifestyle.

DINNER MENU

MONDAY Fiery Chicken-Stuffed Eggplant *p. 134*

TUESDAY Wild Rice and Bok Choy Salad with Peanut Dressing *p. 55*

WEDNESDAY Oven-Roasted Salmon with Fingerling Potatoes *p. 122*

THURSDAY Root Vegetable Shepherd's Pie *p. 150*

FRIDAY Sun-Dried Tomato and Kalamata Olive Linguine *p. 104*

SHODPPING LIST

MEAT AND POULTRY

- ☐ Beef, ground, extra-lean, 1 pound
- ☐ Chicken, ground, 1 pound

SEAFOOD

- ☐ Salmon, boneless, skinless,
  4 (5-ounce) fillets

DAIRY AND DAIRY SUBSTITUTES

- ☐ Parmesan cheese, 1 ounce
- ☐ Yogurt, plain, ¾ cup

PRODUCE AND HERBS

- ☐ Asparagus, 12 spears
- ☐ Basil leaves, 1 bunch
- ☐ Baby bok choy, 8
- ☐ Cabbage, green, 1 head
- ☐ Carrots, 1
- ☐ Cauliflower, 1 head
- ☐ Celeriac, 1
- ☐ Chives, 1 bunch
- ☐ Dill, 1 bunch
- ☐ Eggplants, 2
- ☐ Fingerling potatoes, 1 pound
- ☐ Garlic cloves, 2
- ☐ Garlic, minced, 2 tablespoons
- ☐ Ginger, 2-inch piece
- ☐ Kale, 1 bunch
- ☐ Lemons, 2
- ☐ Oregano, 1 bunch
- ☐ Red bell peppers, 2

- ☐ Scallion, 1
- ☐ Spinach, 1 cup
- ☐ Sweet onions, 2
- ☐ Sweet potatoes, 3
- ☐ Tomato, 1

SPECIAL PANTRY ITEMS

- ☐ Harissa, 2 tablespoons
- ☐ Kalamata olives, ½ cup
- ☐ Pine nuts, 2 tablespoons
- ☐ Sun-dried tomatoes, ½ cup

REGULAR PANTRY ITEMS

- ☐ Apple cider vinegar,
  2 tablespoons
- ☐ Cashews, 2 tablespoons
- ☐ Diced tomatoes, sodium-free,
  1 (28-ounce) can
- ☐ Freshly ground black pepper
- ☐ Garbanzo beans, sodium-free,
  2 (15-ounce) cans
- ☐ Honey, 1 tablespoon
- ☐ Olive oil, ½ cup
- ☐ Peanut butter, natural, ¼ cup
- ☐ Peas, frozen, 1 cup
- ☐ Red pepper flakes
- ☐ Sea salt
- ☐ Tamari, 2 tablespoons
- ☐ Whole-wheat linguine, 8 ounces
- ☐ Wild rice, ½ cup uncooked

Prep Ahead

- The entire Fiery Chicken-Stuffed Eggplant recipe can be assembled.
- Make the dressing for the Wild Rice and Bok Choy Salad with Peanut Dressing.
- Cook the wild rice for the Wild Rice and Bok Choy Salad with Peanut Dressing.
- Blanch the fingerling potatoes for the Oven-Roasted Salmon with Fingerling Potatoes.
- Assemble the entire Oven-Roasted Salmon with Fingerling Potatoes recipe.
- Assemble the entire Root Vegetable Shepherd's Pie recipe.
- Make the pesto for the Sun-Dried Tomato and Kalamata Olive Linguine.
- Cook the linguine for the Sun-Dried Tomato and Kalamata Olive Linguine.

Leftovers

Several of the ingredients needed for the recipes will not be used up entirely. Here are some suggestions for leftover ingredients:

- The basil from the Fiery Chicken-Stuffed Eggplant is also used for the Oven-Roasted Salmon with Fingerling Potatoes.
- Use the leftover cabbage from the Wild Rice and Bok Choy Salad with Peanut Dressing for salads or side dishes.
- The remaining cauliflower (½ head) from the Root Vegetable Shepherd's Pie can be a side dish, soup, stew, or snack.
- Pesto from the Sun-Dried Tomato and Kalamata Olive Linguine is a wonderful spread for sandwiches and a topping for meat and fish.

BEYOND WEEK 3

After Week 3, you will be creating your own meal plans for clean-eating dinners. If you enjoyed effortless planning, you can always repeat the plan again. However, there are many other scrumptious clean-eating dinners, including sides and desserts, to experience in this book. You can also add your own recipes to round out the choices you find here. No matter what strategy you choose to follow, maintaining your clean-eating lifestyle is the ultimate goal.

CLEAN & EASY PORTABLE LUNCHES

Clean-eating dinners are just part of the strategy for successfully adopting this lifestyle. One of the main clean-eating principles is to bring clean-eating foods with you whenever you leave the house, especially for lunch. Try prepping lunch and nutritious snack items and storing them in the refrigerator. Clean-eating lunches should be a satisfying mixture of lean protein, complex carbohydrates, and healthy fats so you can recharge for your afternoon activities.

Here are 10 lunch suggestions to support a clean-eating lifestyle:

1. Leftovers from dinner the evening before such as salads, stews, casseroles, or any other items you want to use up. If you have cooked chicken, fish, or meat, you can create wraps or use the protein as a salad or side topping.

2. Whole-grain sandwiches, wraps, or pitas stuffed with lean protein, eggs, quinoa, vegetables, fruit, feta or goat cheese, or nut butters.

3. Pasta salads or hot pasta dishes topped with diced chicken and heaped with tasty fresh vegetables. Try tossing cold pasta with pesto or tahini and topping it with chopped nuts or feta cheese.

4. Lettuce wraps with grilled or broiled meats, nuts, grains, vegetables, chopped mango or papaya, fresh herbs, and sesame seeds.

5. Composed "bowls" with cooked grains (quinoa, wheat berries, wild rice), avocado, chopped fruit, lots of vegetables, cooked meats or poultry, seeds, nuts, and homemade dressings.

6. Clean-eating sushi with nori, crab or cooked shrimp, shredded vegetables, rice, shredded fruit, nuts, and peanut dipping sauce.

7. Frittata muffins with egg, vegetables, whole-grain pasta, legumes, feta or goat cheese, or chopped cooked chicken. Wrap the grab-and-go muffin in a whole-grain tortilla and serve with fresh fruit.

8. Hearty soups and stews with lots of chopped meats, vegetables, beans, and whole-grain noodles topped with yogurt, seeds, or goat cheese. Add some whole-grain crackers on the side.

9. Savory or sweet oatmeal or whole-grain dishes with nut milks, yogurt, chopped sweet potato or pumpkin, fresh fruit, nuts, seeds, dried fruit, and a drizzle of maple syrup or honey.

10. Heaps of cut vegetables (crudité) with hardboiled eggs, hummus, tahini, or homemade clean-eating dressing. Add whole-grain pita or crackers and some fresh fruit to round out the meal.

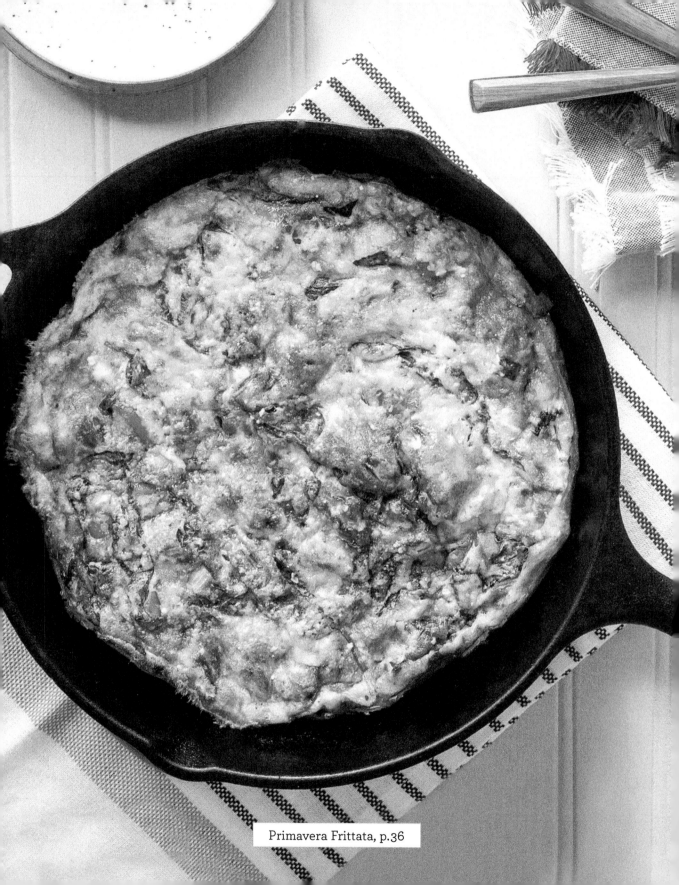

Primavera Frittata, p.36

3

BREAKFAST FOR DINNER

FRIED EGG SQUASH CIRCLES

Gluten-Free • Dairy-Free • Nut-Free • Vegetarian

SERVES 4

PREP: 5 minutes

COOK: 25 minutes

1 butternut squash,
cut crosswise into ½-inch
slices and seeded

1 tablespoon olive oil

8 eggs

Sea salt

Freshly ground
black pepper

Pinch sweet paprika

2 tablespoons chopped
fresh parsley

Producing hundreds of breakfast plates in a few hours requires a careful hand on the flat-top grill and a little device called an egg ring. Eggs are cracked into the ring and it corrals the whites, so the finished product is compact. Egg rings can be expensive, so I use cooked squash and pepper rings to do the same job for a fraction of the cost. The best part is that you can eat the squash along with the perfectly fried eggs.

1. Preheat the oven to 400°F. Line a baking sheet with parchment paper and set aside.

2. Lightly oil the squash slices with the olive oil.

3. Place the squash slices on the baking sheet and bake until just cooked, about 15 minutes.

4. Crack an egg in the center of each slice and sprinkle with sea salt, pepper, and paprika.

5. Bake in the oven until the eggs are set, about 10 minutes.

6. Top with the parsley and serve.

ON THE SIDE: Avocado Chopped Salad (page 47)

PREP TIP: The squash can be cooked ahead of time and stored in the refrigerator, wrapped in plastic wrap, for up to three days. Take the squash out and let it come to room temperature before continuing with the recipe from Step 4.

Per Serving: Calories: 220; Fat: 12g; Protein: 13g; Total Carbs: 17g; Fiber: 4g; Sodium: 188mg

BEAN AND EGG TACOS

Dairy-Free • Nut-Free • Vegetarian • Kids Love It

SERVES 4

PREP: 15 minutes

COOK: 5 minutes

1 cup canned black beans, sodium-free

1 teaspoon olive oil

6 large eggs, beaten

4 whole-grain or corn taco shells

½ cup tomato salsa

½ avocado, diced

2 tablespoons chopped fresh cilantro

1 cup shredded lettuce

Huevos rancheros, basically a tortilla-wrapped breakfast "sandwich," is usually the first thing to come to mind when considering a Southwestern-themed egg dish, but taco shells work well, too. Tacos are always a huge hit because they are festive and a little messy depending on the stuffing. If you want a neater meal, substitute whole-grain tortillas and roll them up.

1. Place a small saucepan over low-medium heat and add the black beans. Cook until warmed, about 5 minutes.

2. While that cooks, place a medium skillet over medium-high heat and add the olive oil.

3. Add the eggs to the skillet. Cook, scrambling, for about 5 minutes, or until they are fluffy, cooked through, and dry.

4. Evenly divide the egg mixture among the taco shells.

5. Top each taco with the black beans, salsa, avocado, cilantro, and lettuce. Serve immediately.

ON THE SIDE: Fresh fruit

VARIATION TIP: For a little heat, add chopped, fresh jalapeño peppers or a splash of hot sauce. You can also use hot salsa in the same amount as indicated in the recipe.

Per Serving: Calories: 347; Fat: 19g; Protein: 16g; Total Carbs: 33g; Fiber: 12g; Sodium: 487mg

VEGGIE EGG WRAP

Dairy-Free • Nut-Free • Vegetarian

SERVES 4

PREP: 10 minutes

COOK: 10 minutes

1 tablespoon olive oil

8 eggs, beaten

¼ sweet onion, chopped

½ red bell pepper, chopped

½ carrot, grated

½ cup chopped cauliflower

1 cup chopped kale

1 teaspoon minced garlic

1 teaspoon chopped fresh basil

1 teaspoon chopped fresh oregano

4 (10-inch) whole-wheat tortillas

Eggs are fantastic for dinner because they take very little time to make, are usually in your refrigerator anyway, and are extremely healthy. Eggs contain 6 grams of high-quality protein and 14 important nutrients such as iron, choline, and vitamins A, D, and E. Eggs are also a great source of omega-3 fatty acids to help protect the heart and support brain health.

1. Place a large skillet over medium-high heat and add the olive oil.

2. In a large bowl, whisk together the eggs, sweet onion, red bell pepper, carrot, cauliflower, kale, garlic, basil, and oregano.

3. Pour the egg mixture into the skillet and cook until the egg is set, lifting the edges to let any uncooked egg flow underneath, about 10 minutes.

4. Lay the tortillas on a clean work surface. Cut the cooked eggs into 4 pieces and place 1 piece on each tortilla.

5. Working with one tortilla at a time, fold the sides in over the filling. Then fold the bottom up over the filling and continue rolling the tortilla into a tight cylinder. Serve.

ON THE SIDE: Sliced tomatoes

PREP TIP: You can use leftover cooked vegetables such as cauliflower or carrots in this dish. Or, if you prefer, you can blanch these veggies to create a softer texture.

Per Serving: Calories: 300; Fat: 14g; Protein: 15g; Total Carbs: 26g; Fiber: 3g; Sodium: 440mg

PRIMAVERA FRITTATA

Gluten-Free · Vegetarian · Kids Love It

SERVES 4

PREP: 10 minutes

COOK: 20 minutes

1 tablespoon olive oil

¼ sweet onion, chopped

2 teaspoons minced garlic

1 small carrot, grated

1 zucchini, diced

½ red bell pepper, diced

1 sweet potato, diced

1 cup baby spinach

8 large eggs, beaten

¼ cup unsweetened almond milk

½ teaspoon ground cumin

½ teaspoon ground coriander

½ cup crumbled goat cheese

Sea salt

Freshly ground black pepper

One of my duties in my first restaurant job was to make quiches for the lunch and light dinner menus. This taught me the art of the perfect pie crust, but it was time-consuming and fraught with the possibility of failure. Imagine my delight when I discovered frittatas—basically a crustless quiche! Even an amateur cook can master this culinary creation with little effort.

1. Preheat the oven to 425°F.

2. Place a large ovenproof skillet over medium-high heat. Add the olive oil.

3. Sauté the sweet onion and garlic until softened, about 3 minutes.

4. Stir in the carrot, zucchini, red bell pepper, sweet potato, and spinach and sauté until the vegetables are tender, about 5 minutes.

5. In a medium bowl, whisk together the eggs, almond milk, cumin, and coriander.

6. Pour the eggs into the skillet and sprinkle with the goat cheese.

7. Cook the frittata on the stove until the eggs are almost cooked through and set, lifting the edges to let the raw egg flow underneath, about 10 minutes.

8. Place the skillet in the preheated oven. Bake the frittata until the top is set, about 5 minutes.

9. Remove from the oven and let stand for 5 minutes.

10. Season with sea salt and pepper. Cut into quarters and serve.

ON THE SIDE: Serve with a fresh green salad

LEFTOVERS TIP: Frittatas are delicious both hot and cold, so store any extras in the refrigerator and wrap a chunk in a multigrain tortilla for breakfast. Add a little chopped tomato and shredded lettuce or a splash of hot sauce.

Per Serving: Calories: 290; Fat: 19g; Protein: 19g; Total Carbs: 13g; Fiber: 2g; Sodium: 255mg

BROCCOLI–BROWN RICE EGG MUFFINS

Gluten-Free • Nut-Free • Vegetarian

SERVES 4

PREP: 10 minutes

COOK: 20 minutes

Nonstick cooking spray

8 eggs

1 cup ricotta

1 scallion, white and green parts, chopped

1 tablespoon chopped fresh parsley

Pinch red pepper flakes

1 cup cooked brown basmati rice

1 cup chopped blanched broccoli

Savory muffins are easy to make and very convenient when you need a quick grab-and-go meal for an activity-packed evening. Brown rice adds substance and texture to the muffins along with a pleasing, almost nutty flavor. Other whole grains, such as quinoa, bulgur, or wheat berries, could also work beautifully.

1. Preheat the oven to 350°F and spray 12 muffin cups with the cooking spray.

2. In a large bowl, whisk together the eggs, ricotta, scallion, parsley, and red pepper flakes.

3. Evenly divide the rice and broccoli between the muffin cups.

4. Fill the muffin cups with the egg mixture.

5. Bake until the muffins are golden and the eggs are set, about 20 minutes. Serve.

ON THE SIDE: 1 slice whole-grain toast

LEFTOVERS TIP: Wrap the egg muffins individually in plastic wrap after they are completely cooled and store them for three days in the refrigerator or one month in the freezer.

Per Serving: Calories: 238; Fat: 14g; Protein: 19g; Total Carbs: 10g; Fiber: 2g; Sodium: 172mg

EGG-TOPPED LENTIL BOWL WITH SPINACH

Gluten-Free • Nut-Free • Vegetarian

SERVES 4

PREP: 10 minutes

COOK: 20 minutes

2 tablespoons olive
oil, divided

½ sweet onion, chopped

1 teaspoon minced garlic

1 cup chopped cauliflower

1 cup baby spinach

2 cups cooked red lentils

1 cup cherry
tomatoes, halved

1 tablespoon chopped
fresh basil

4 eggs

½ cup low-sodium
feta cheese

I am partial to red or brown lentils because I find the green variety a little unattractive in most recipes. Make sure the lentils in this dish retain their shape and texture, rather than going to mush, so that the egg yolk can drip through the other ingredients when it is broken.

1. Place a large skillet over medium-high heat and add 1 tablespoon of the olive oil.

2. Sauté the sweet onion and garlic until softened, about 3 minutes.

3. Add the cauliflower and spinach. Sauté until the cauliflower is tender and the spinach wilts, about 4 minutes.

4. Stir in the lentils, tomatoes, and basil and reduce the heat to low. Cook until the lentils are heated through, stirring occasionally, about 5 minutes.

5. Spoon the lentil mixture into 4 bowls and wipe out the skillet.

6. Add the remaining olive oil to the skillet, and increase the heat to medium-high. Fry the eggs until the whites are set, about 5 minutes.

7. Use a spatula to place 1 egg on each lentil bowl. Top each bowl with feta cheese and serve.

ON THE SIDE: 1 slice whole-grain toast

SUBSTITUTION TIP: Instead of topping the lentil bowl with fried eggs, push the lentils over to the side of the skillet and scramble the eggs in the empty space. Stir the scrambled eggs into the lentil mixture and serve.

Per Serving: Calories: 298; Fat: 14g; Protein: 18g; Total Carbs: 26g; Fiber: 10g; Sodium: 271mg

COTTAGE CHEESE EGG BAKE

Gluten-Free • Nut-Free • Vegetarian • Kids Love It

SERVES 4

PREP: 10 minutes

COOK: 20 minutes

Olive oil, for greasing
the baking dish

8 eggs

1 cup cottage cheese

1 cup chopped baby
spinach

1 teaspoon minced garlic

Sea salt

Freshly ground
black pepper

1 cup halved cherry
tomatoes

½ cup diced roasted
red bell pepper

1 scallion, white and
green parts, chopped

This dish is one of my favorite time-saving choices midweek when everyone is going in different directions but still needs to fill up. I put it together in the morning between cups of coffee and pop it in the oven right when I get home. By the time I have fed the dogs and changed into my comfy clothes, dinner is on the table.

1. Preheat the oven to 350°F. Lightly grease an 8-by-8-inch baking dish with the olive oil and set aside.

2. In a medium bowl, stir together the eggs, cottage cheese, spinach, and garlic.

3. Season the egg mixture with sea salt and pepper.

4. Spread the tomatoes, roasted red bell pepper, and scallion in the baking dish.

5. Pour the egg mixture over the vegetables.

6. Bake the eggs until just set and lightly browned, about 20 minutes. Serve.

ON THE SIDE: Grapefruit halves

PREP TIP: There are many good-quality roasted-red-pepper products in jars or cans if you do not want to roast your own. Look for peppers with very few ingredients and watch the sodium content.

Per Serving: Calories: 191; Fat: 10g; Protein: 20g; Total Carbs: 6g; Fiber: 1g; Sodium: 438mg

SWEET-POTATO HARVEST PANCAKES

Vegetarian • Kids Love It

SERVES 4

PREP: 10 minutes

COOK: 18 minutes

1 cup whole-wheat flour

1 cup almond flour

2 teaspoons baking powder

1 teaspoon ground cinnamon

½ teaspoon ground ginger

¼ teaspoon ground nutmeg

½ teaspoon baking soda

Pinch sea salt

1 cup mashed cooked sweet potato

1 cup unsweetened almond milk

½ cup plain yogurt

2 eggs

¼ cup maple syrup

1 teaspoon pure vanilla extract

1½ tablespoons melted coconut oil

My children are now 18 and 15, but still ask for pancakes at dinnertime every few weeks. It is an incredibly easy meal to prepare, and a stack of golden, fragrant pancakes is the ultimate comfort food after a long day at work or school. Drizzle them with maple syrup or try a scattering of chopped, toasted pecans for extra flavor and texture.

1. In a large bowl, stir together the whole-wheat flour, almond flour, baking powder, cinnamon, ginger, nutmeg, baking soda, and sea salt.

2. In a medium bowl, stir together the sweet potato, almond milk, yogurt, eggs, maple syrup, and vanilla until just combined.

3. Place a large skillet over medium-high heat and add 1½ teaspoons of the coconut oil.

4. Pour the batter into the skillet, about ⅓ cup for each pancake, and spread it out a little with the back of a spoon.

5. Cook the pancakes until golden brown on the bottom, then flip and cook the opposite side until golden, about 6 minutes total.

6. Repeat Steps 4 and 5 until all of the batter has been used and you have 12 pancakes.

7. Serve.

ON THE SIDE: Fresh fruit

LEFTOVERS TIP: Wrap the chilled pancakes in plastic wrap and store them for up to two days in the refrigerator. For a delightful snack, create a cold pancake wrap with nut butter and sliced bananas.

Per Serving (3 pancakes): Calories: 376; Fat: 10g; Protein: 10g; Total Carbs: 56g; Fiber: 5g; Sodium: 305mg

SWEET OATMEAL BAKE

Gluten-Free • Dairy-Free • Vegetarian • Kids Love It

SERVES 6

PREP: 5 minutes

COOK: 30 minutes

Coconut oil, for greasing the baking dish

2 apples, peeled, cored, and diced

2½ cups gluten-free rolled oats

¼ cup chopped pecans

1 teaspoon baking powder

1 teaspoon ground cinnamon

½ teaspoon ground nutmeg

¼ teaspoon sea salt

2 cups unsweetened almond milk

½ cup maple syrup

2 eggs

1 teaspoon pure vanilla extract

Oatmeal is incredibly easy to prepare, but sometimes the 10 minutes spent stirring this grain on the stove takes too much time in the morning. Baked oatmeal is the perfect solution when you're craving a simple meal.

1. Preheat the oven to 350°F. Grease an 8-by-8-inch baking dish with the coconut oil and arrange the apple pieces evenly on the bottom.

2. In a medium bowl, combine the oats, pecans, baking powder, cinnamon, nutmeg, and sea salt. Mix well.

3. In a small bowl, whisk together the almond milk, maple syrup, eggs, and vanilla.

4. Add the almond-milk mixture to the oat mixture and stir to combine.

5. Pour the oatmeal mixture over the apples and spread evenly.

6. Bake until the top is golden and the oatmeal is set firm, about 30 minutes. Serve.

ON THE SIDE: Fresh fruit or plain yogurt

PREP TIP: The entire recipe can be prepared the day before and kept in the refrigerator, covered, until you wish to serve this dish. Place the casserole in a 350°F oven and bake for 30 minutes.

Per Serving: Calories: 270; Fat: 12g; Protein: 5g; Total Carbs: 39g; Fiber: 5g; Sodium: 154mg

COCONUT FRENCH TOAST
WITH BERRIES

Dairy-Free • Vegetarian • Kids Love It

SERVES 4

PREP: 10 minutes

COOK: 10 minutes

4 eggs

1 cup unsweetened coconut milk

1 tablespoon pure vanilla extract

1 teaspoon ground cinnamon

⅛ teaspoon ground ginger

Pinch ground nutmeg

8 slices multigrain bread

Coconut oil, for greasing the skillet

2 cups mixed fresh berries, your preference

½ cup unsweetened shredded coconut

I adore French toast. It is my request for every Mother's Day and birthday, if someone offers to cook something for me. The coconut adds crunch and a pleasing flavor to the golden bread, creating a dessert-like meal. You can top the pieces with a drizzle of maple syrup, but I find the fresh fruit adds just the right touch of sweetness.

1. In a large bowl, whisk together the eggs, coconut milk, vanilla, cinnamon, ginger, and nutmeg until blended.

2. Dredge 4 bread slices in the egg mixture and shake off any excess.

3. Preheat a large nonstick skillet over medium heat and brush it with coconut oil.

4. Place the bread slices in the skillet and cook until lightly browned, about 3 minutes.

5. Flip the bread slices over and cook the other side for 2 minutes. Remove from the pan to a plate to keep warm (cover lightly with aluminum foil).

6. Wipe the skillet out with paper towel and cook the remaining bread slices.

7. Serve warm, sprinkled with berries and coconut.

ON THE SIDE: Serve with plain yogurt

VARIATION TIP: Try maple or almond extract or freshly squeezed orange juice to flavor the egg mixture. If you use the other extracts, top with sliced almonds instead of coconut.

Per Serving: Calories: 328; Fat: 27g; Protein: 9g; Total Carbs: 31g; Fiber: 6g; Sodium: 72mg

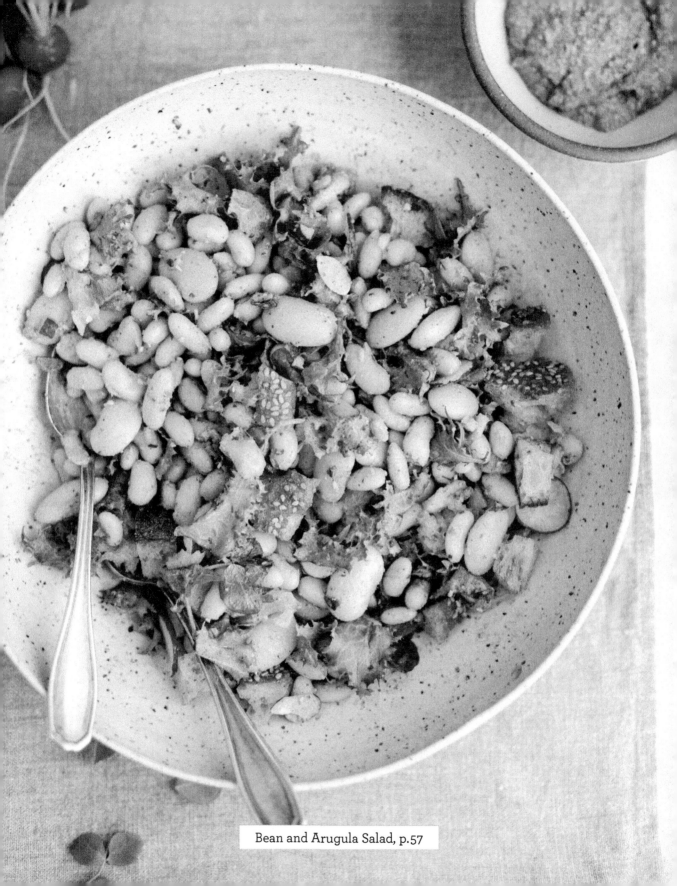

Bean and Arugula Salad, p.57

4

SALADS

AVOCADO CHOPPED SALAD

Gluten-Free • Vegetarian • Kids Love It

SERVES 4

PREP: 15 minutes

COOK: 0 minutes

FOR THE DRESSING

¼ cup olive oil

3 tablespoons white
wine vinegar

2 teaspoons Dijon mustard

2 teaspoons honey

1 teaspoon minced garlic

Sea salt

Freshly ground
black pepper

FOR THE SALAD

4 cups baby spinach

2 cups shredded kale

1 English cucumber, diced

1 avocado, peeled, pitted,
and diced

1 cup green beans, trimmed
and cut into 1-inch pieces

¼ cup chopped pistachios

¼ cup crumbled
goat cheese

1 scallion, white and green
parts, chopped

Chopped salads are similar to regular salads, but the ingredients are cut into uniform pieces to create a composed look. This recipe is a visual feast of greens and whites, with almost every shade covered in a delicious plateful. If spring could be captured in one dish, this would be a pretty good representation of the season.

TO MAKE THE DRESSING

1. In a small bowl, whisk together the olive oil, vinegar, mustard, honey, and garlic.

2. Season with sea salt and pepper.

3. Set aside.

TO MAKE THE SALAD

1. In a large bowl, toss together the spinach, kale, cucumber, avocado, green beans, and pistachios.

2. Add the dressing and toss.

3. Serve topped with goat cheese and scallion.

ON THE SIDE: Quinoa Salad–Stuffed Pita (page 69)

PREP TIP: You can certainly buy shelled pistachios because it saves time and is easier, but this product can be very expensive. Get a bag of unshelled nuts and shell them yourself, saving the extra for a nice snack.

Per Serving: Calories: 323; Fat: 26g; Protein: 7g; Total Carbs: 18g; Fiber: 6g; Sodium: 110mg

BROCCOLI-ALMOND SLAW

Gluten-Free • Vegetarian • Kids Love It

SERVES 4

PREP: 20 minutes

COOK: 0 minutes

FOR THE DRESSING

¼ cup plain yogurt

3 tablespoons freshly squeezed orange juice

1 tablespoon apple cider vinegar

1 teaspoon maple syrup

1 teaspoon chopped fresh oregano

Sea salt

Freshly ground black pepper

FOR THE SALAD

1 head broccoli

2 carrots, shredded

1 parsnip, shredded

1 scallion, white and green parts, chopped

¼ cup dried cranberries

¼ cup sliced almonds

Coleslaw has a bit of a reputation of being boring and bland, but this salad bursts with flavor, and the brightly colored carrots and cranberries create a gorgeous presentation. If you want to add cabbage to the mix, it combines well with the other ingredients. Only throw in 1 cup of shredded cabbage so it doesn't overwhelm the other vegetables.

TO MAKE THE DRESSING

1. In a small bowl, whisk together the yogurt, orange juice, vinegar, maple syrup, and oregano.

2. Season the dressing with sea salt and pepper.

3. Set aside.

TO MAKE THE SALAD

1. Cut the broccoli into small florets and grate the stalks. Transfer the florets and the grated stalks to a large bowl.

2. Add the carrots, parsnip, scallion, cranberries, and almonds to the broccoli.

3. Add the dressing and toss to coat.

4. Serve.

ON THE SIDE: Turkey Breast and Mango Sandwich with Avocado (page 70)

SUBSTITUTION TIP: To save time, use a prepackaged broccoli slaw, one that contains carrots and broccoli. This is simpler, but won't include any tasty broccoli florets that add bulk and texture to the dish.

Per Serving: Calories: 130; Fat: 4g; Protein: 6g; Total Carbs: 21g; Fiber: 7g; Sodium: 146mg

BLUEBERRY-AVOCADO SPINACH SALAD

Gluten-Free • Dairy-Free • Vegan • Vegetarian • Kids Love It

SERVES 4

PREP: 20 minutes

COOK: 0 minutes

FOR THE DRESSING

¼ cup olive oil

2 tablespoons balsamic vinegar

2 tablespoons maple syrup

Sea salt

Freshly ground black pepper

FOR THE SALAD

4 cups spinach

2 cups cooked bulgur

2 cups blueberries

1 avocado, peeled, pitted, and diced

½ jicama, peeled and shredded

½ cup chopped hazelnuts

The colors and textures of this salad are exceptional. Creamy jicama, vibrant blueberries, pastel avocados, and deep-green spinach drizzled with luscious maple-spiked dressing is an inspired choice for a light dinner. Blueberries are low on the glycemic index while being high in fiber and antioxidants. Jicama looks a little like a potato but has crisp, mild flesh similar to an Asian pear. Jicama is a wonderful source of vitamin C and is fat-free, so it makes a great snack when you need an energy lift.

TO MAKE THE DRESSING

1. In a small bowl, whisk together the olive oil, balsamic vinegar, and maple syrup.

2. Season with sea salt and pepper.

3. Set aside.

TO MAKE THE SALAD

1. In a large bowl, toss together the spinach, bulgur, blueberries, avocado, jicama, and hazelnuts.

2. Add the dressing and toss to combine.

3. Serve.

ON THE SIDE: Broccoli-Kale Soup (page 62)

LEFTOVERS TIP: The other half of the jicama can be added to salads, soups, stews, and side dishes. Brush the cut edge of the jicama with lemon juice and store in a sealed plastic bag.

Per Serving: Calories: 445; Fat: 27g; Protein: 6g; Total Carbs: 47g; Fiber: 14g; Sodium: 136mg

FENNEL-TOMATO SALAD WITH SHRIMP

Gluten-Free • Dairy-Free • Nut-Free

SERVES 4

PREP: 15 minutes

COOK: 15 minutes

FOR THE DRESSING

¼ cup olive oil

2 tablespoons apple cider vinegar

1 teaspoon Dijon mustard

1 teaspoon chopped fresh basil

Sea salt

Freshly ground black pepper

FOR THE SALAD

2 cups halved cherry tomatoes

½ bulb fennel, thinly sliced

½ English cucumber, cut in half lengthwise and thinly sliced

4 cups chopped baby kale

1 scallion, white and green parts, chopped

1 pound cooked shrimp, peeled and deveined

Fennel is a pretty vegetable from the same family as carrots, dill, and parsley, with frothy fronds and an elegant shape. Eating fennel regularly can help control blood sugar and lower cholesterol. The other half of the fennel bulb left after making this salad can be sautéed as a delightful side dish.

TO MAKE THE DRESSING

1. In a small bowl, whisk together the olive oil, vinegar, mustard, and basil.

2. Season the dressing with sea salt and pepper.

3. Set aside.

TO MAKE THE SALAD

1. In a large bowl, toss together the cherry tomatoes, fennel, cucumber, kale, and scallion with ¾ of the dressing.

2. Arrange the salad on 4 plates and top evenly with the shrimp.

3. Drizzle the salad with the remaining dressing and serve.

ON THE SIDE: Whole-Grain Penne with Spinach Pesto (page 88)

PREP TIP: If you have some extra time to make dinner, use fresh shrimp instead of cooked, so you can grill and broil it for extra flavor. Season the shrimp lightly with garlic powder before cooking.

Per Serving: Calories: 310; Fat: 14g; Protein: 29g; Total Carbs: 16g; Fiber: 3g; Sodium: 395mg

MILLET-PISTACHIO SALAD WITH PEACHES

Gluten-Free • Dairy-Free • Vegetarian

SERVES 4

PREP: 20 minutes

COOK: 0 minutes

FOR THE DRESSING

3 tablespoons olive oil

3 tablespoons freshly squeezed orange juice

1 tablespoon honey

1 tablespoon tahini

Sea salt

Freshly ground black pepper

FOR THE SALAD

4 cups mixed greens

1 cup cooked millet

1 (15-ounce) can garbanzo beans, drained and rinsed

1 red bell pepper, thinly sliced

2 peaches, pitted and sliced

½ cup toasted pistachios

1 scallion, white and green parts, chopped

Millet is an underutilized ancient grain that has been a staple for more than 10,000 years in India and Asia, but it is not common in North America. Packed with nutrition, this gluten-free grain contains protein, fiber, choline, magnesium, potassium, phosphorus, and zinc. It's also heart-friendly, helps stabilize blood sugar, and can help protect against cataracts and gallstones.

TO MAKE THE DRESSING

1. In a small bowl, whisk together the olive oil, orange juice, honey, and tahini.

2. Season the dressing with sea salt and pepper.

3. Set aside.

TO MAKE THE SALAD

1. In a large bowl, toss together the greens, millet, garbanzo beans, red bell pepper, peaches, pistachios, scallion, and salad dressing.

2. Serve.

ON THE SIDE: Chicken and Sun-Dried Tomato Wraps (page 71)

VARIATION TIP: Top the salad with grilled chicken, shrimp, or a nice piece of broiled fish to create a more substantial meal. This extra protein can be added hot or cold.

Per Serving: Calories: 478; Fat: 19g; Protein: 14g; Total Carbs: 59g; Fiber: 13g; Sodium: 177mg

SOUTHWESTERN COUSCOUS SALAD WITH LIME DRESSING

Nut-Free • Vegetarian • Kids Love It

SERVES 4

PREP: 15 minutes

COOK: 0 minutes

FOR THE DRESSING

¼ cup freshly squeezed lime juice

1 tablespoon honey

½ teaspoon ground cumin

Pinch chili powder

¼ cup olive oil

Sea salt

Freshly ground black pepper

Couscous was a culinary revelation for me when I first started cooking in North Africa—I initially thought this versatile ingredient was a grain, rather than a pasta. The ease of preparation is one of its best features; if you can boil water, you can make couscous. Look for whole-wheat products to avoid white flour in your diet.

TO MAKE THE DRESSING

1. In a small bowl, whisk together the lime juice, honey, cumin, and chili powder.

2. Whisk in the olive oil until it is emulsified, and season with sea salt and pepper.

3. Set aside.

FOR THE SALAD

1 cup cooked Israeli couscous

1 (15-ounce) can sodium-free black beans, drained and rinsed

1 red bell pepper, chopped

1 scallion, white and green parts, chopped

½ avocado, peeled, pitted, and chopped

5 cups baby spinach

¼ cup low-sodium feta cheese

2 tablespoons chopped fresh cilantro

TO MAKE THE SALAD

1. In a medium bowl, stir together the couscous, black beans, red bell pepper, scallion, avocado, and half of the dressing.

2. Arrange the spinach on 4 plates and drizzle with the remaining dressing.

3. Top the spinach with the couscous mixture, feta cheese, and cilantro.

4. Serve.

ON THE SIDE: Chicken and Sun-Dried Tomato Wraps (page 71)

VARIATION TIP: Wheat berries, bulgur, brown rice, or quinoa can replace the couscous if you prefer those ingredients more than the pasta. Use the same amount and prepare the recipe the same way.

Per Serving: Calories: 418; Fat: 19g; Protein: 14g; Total Carbs: 48g; Fiber: 12g; Sodium: 167mg

SOBA NOODLE AND CARROT SALAD

Dairy-Free • Nut-Free • Vegetarian • Kids Love It

SERVES 4

PREP: 25 minutes

COOK: 0 minutes

FOR THE DRESSING

2 tablespoons olive oil

2 tablespoons sesame oil

2 tablespoons tamari

2 tablespoons freshly squeezed lime juice

1 tablespoon honey

1 tablespoon freshly grated ginger

Pinch red pepper flakes

FOR THE SALAD

4 cups cooked soba noodles

4 carrots, peeled into long ribbons with a vegetable peeler

1 zucchini, cut into long ribbons with a vegetable peeler

2 cups shredded bok choy

1 cup julienned snow peas

2 tablespoons chopped fresh cilantro

2 tablespoons toasted sesame seeds

If your clean-eating plan is very strict, you'll have to source the soba noodles for this dish carefully. Some products contain white flour rather than just buckwheat, so read the labels and look for dark, grayish-brown noodles. Pure soba noodles could be easier to find in Asian markets rather than your local grocery store.

TO MAKE THE DRESSING

1. In a small bowl, whisk together the olive oil, sesame oil, tamari, lime juice, honey, ginger, and red pepper flakes.

2. Set aside.

TO MAKE THE SALAD

1. In a large bowl, toss together the noodles, carrots, zucchini, bok choy, snow peas, cilantro, and salad dressing.

2. Serve topped with sesame seeds.

ON THE SIDE: Beef-Broccoli Stir-Fry (page 148)

PREP TIP: If you prepare lots of vegetable noodles, add a mandolin or spiralizer to your kitchen tools. These devices can create sliced, julienned, and spiralized vegetables and fruits easily.

Per Serving: Calories: 336; Fat: 15g; Protein: 10g; Total Carbs: 42g; Fiber: 5g; Sodium: 653mg

WILD RICE AND BOK CHOY SALAD WITH PEANUT DRESSING

Gluten-Free • Dairy-Free • Vegetarian

MEAL PLAN
WEEK 3
TUESDAY

SERVES 4

PREP: 25 minutes

COOK: 0 minutes

FOR THE DRESSING

¼ cup natural peanut butter

2 tablespoons apple cider vinegar

2 tablespoons tamari

1 tablespoon honey

2 teaspoons freshly grated ginger

1 to 2 tablespoons water, to thin

FOR THE SALAD

2 cups shredded bok choy

2 cups shredded green cabbage

1 cup cooked wild rice

1 cup grated carrots

1 red bell pepper, diced

¼ cup chopped fresh cilantro

1 scallion, white and green parts, chopped

2 tablespoons chopped cashews

Wild rice, an aquatic grass, is an indigenous plant where I live in Northern Ontario, and a family favorite. It grows naturally in sparkling lakes without pesticides or fertilizers, reseeding itself. Wild rice is gluten-free, high in protein and fiber, and a terrific source of lysine, B vitamins, potassium, and phosphorous.

TO MAKE THE DRESSING

1. In a small bowl, whisk together the peanut butter, vinegar, tamari, honey, and ginger.

2. Add the water to thin the dressing to the desired consistency.

3. Set aside.

TO MAKE THE SALAD

1. In a large bowl, toss together the bok choy, cabbage, wild rice, carrots, red bell pepper, cilantro, and scallion.

2. Add the dressing and toss to coat.

3. Serve topped with cashews.

ON THE SIDE: Turkey Breast and Mango Sandwich with Avocado (page 70)

PREP TIP: Wild rice will keep in the refrigerator in a sealed container for up to five days, as long as you cool it completely before covering. Cooking the rice ahead will save time on the day you wish to serve this salad.

Per Serving: Calories: 331; Fat: 10g; Protein: 14g; Total Carbs: 48g; Fiber: 6g; Sodium: 186mg

ASIAN CHICKEN KALE SALAD

Gluten-Free • Dairy-Free • Kids Love It

SERVES 4

PREP: 20 minutes

COOK: 0 minutes

FOR THE DRESSING

½ cup freshly squeezed lime juice

2 tablespoons tamari

2 tablespoons sweet red chili sauce

2 tablespoons natural peanut butter

1 teaspoon chopped cilantro

FOR THE SALAD

4 cups chopped kale

2 cups shredded baby bok choy

1 cup julienned snow peas

1 red bell pepper, cut into thin strips

1 mango, peeled, pitted, and diced

2 cooked chicken breasts, chopped

¼ cup chopped peanuts

2 tablespoons chopped fresh basil

My mother was of Indonesian and Dutch heritage, so incredibly complex, spicy foods were the norm in my house. When other children in grade school dipped French fries in ketchup, I was enjoying fiery peanut sauce. If you want a milder version of this dressing, cut back on the amount of chili sauce.

TO MAKE THE DRESSING

1. In a small bowl, whisk together the lime juice, tamari, red chili sauce, peanut butter, and cilantro until smooth.

2. Set aside.

TO MAKE THE SALAD

1. In a large bowl, toss together the kale, bok choy, snow peas, red bell pepper, mango, and chicken.

2. Add the dressing and toss to coat.

3. Serve topped with peanuts and basil.

ON THE SIDE: Watermelon Gazpacho (page 61)

PREP TIP: This salad is a great way to use up leftover chicken or turkey if you roast a whole bird. Simply save the extra in plastic bags in the refrigerator or freezer.

Per Serving: Calories: 368; Fat: 14g; Protein: 31g; Total Carbs: 32g; Fiber: 6g; Sodium: 278mg

BEAN AND ARUGULA SALAD

Gluten-Free • Dairy-Free • Nut-Free • Vegan • Vegetarian

SERVES 4

PREP: 20 minutes

COOK: 0 minutes

2 (15-ounce) cans sodium-free navy beans, drained and rinsed

1 (15-ounce) can sodium-free white kidney beans, drained and rinsed

3 cups torn arugula

1 cup sliced radish

½ red onion, chopped

2 tablespoons olive oil

2 tablespoons apple cider vinegar

2 tablespoons chopped fresh parsley

1 tablespoon honey

1 cup whole-grain sesame croutons

My Nana made a bean salad that was famous in her neck of the woods, winning several ribbons at local fairs, and her recipe became a bit of a family secret. This version is as close as I can get from deciphering a page of her kitchen notebook, as faded ink and water damage have erased some quantities and one ingredient. It is still delicious despite any errors!

1. In a large bowl, toss together the navy beans, kidney beans, arugula, radish, red onion, olive oil, vinegar, parsley, and honey until well mixed.

2. Toss in the croutons.

3. Serve.

ON THE SIDE: Creamy Tomato Soup (page 67)

PREP TIP: This salad tastes even better the next day, so prepare it a couple of days in advance and store it in the refrigerator in a covered container. Leave out the croutons until you are ready to serve or they will be soggy.

Per Serving: Calories: 417; Fat: 13g; Protein: 18g; Total Carbs: 56g; Fiber: 18g; Sodium: 79mg

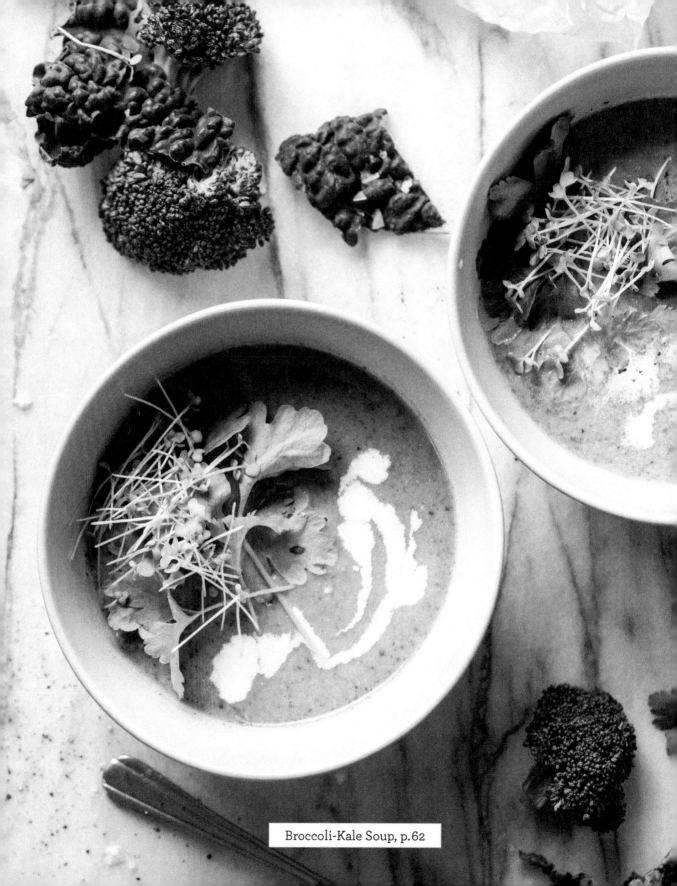

Broccoli-Kale Soup, p.62

5

SOUPS AND SANDWICHES

WATERMELON GAZPACHO

Gluten-Free • Dairy-Free • Nut-Free • Vegan • Vegetarian • Kids Love It

SERVES 4

PREP: 25 minutes

COOK: 0 minutes

1 (4-pound) watermelon, rind removed, diced

2 tablespoons apple cider vinegar

2 shallots, chopped

3 tablespoons chopped fresh basil

Sea salt

1 English cucumber, peeled and finely diced

1 red bell pepper, finely diced

1 tablespoon chopped fresh mint

This novel soup, brimming with sweetness, is a hit with kids. Ripe summer watermelons combine with red bell peppers to create a glorious deep-pink dish. Include a bit of the pale-green flesh under the peel in your soup, as this area has the greatest concentration of disease-fighting phytonutrients.

1. In a food processor or blender, purée the watermelon, vinegar, shallots, and basil until smooth.

2. Transfer the mixture to a large bowl and season with sea salt.

3. Stir in the cucumber and red bell pepper, and chill in the refrigerator.

4. Serve topped with fresh mint.

ON THE SIDE: Broccoli-Almond Slaw (page 48)

PREP TIP: Choose a watermelon that is dark green and has a creamy beige spot to ensure the melon is ripe and juicy. It should feel heavier than its size and be free of soft spots or cracks.

Per Serving: Calories: 163; Fat: 1g; Protein: 4g; Total Carbs: 40g; Fiber: 3g; Sodium: 68mg

BROCCOLI-KALE SOUP

Gluten-Free • Nut-Free • Vegetarian

SERVES 4

PREP: 10 minutes

COOK: 20 minutes

1 tablespoon olive oil

1 sweet onion, chopped

2 celery stalks, sliced

1 teaspoon minced garlic

1 broccoli head, chopped

8 cups sodium-free
vegetable broth

2 tablespoons freshly
squeezed lemon juice

2 cups shredded kale

1 tablespoon chopped
fresh basil

Sea salt

Freshly ground
black pepper

¼ cup plain yogurt,
for garnish

Fresh herbs, sprouts,
or greens, for garnish

Most soups in North America are served piping hot, but cold soups can be refreshing and elegant. This soup is delightful either hot or cold, so you get to choose which temperature suits the occasion. For a truly elegant look, garnish the soup with fresh broccoli sprouts and swirl the yogurt topping with a knife to create a decorative pattern.

1. Place a large saucepan over medium-high heat and add the olive oil.

2. Sauté the sweet onion, celery, and garlic until softened, about 3 minutes.

3. Add the broccoli, vegetable broth, and lemon juice and bring the soup to a boil.

4. Reduce the heat to low and simmer until the broccoli is tender, about 15 minutes.

5. Stir in the kale and basil in the last 5 minutes of cooking time.

6. Transfer the soup to a food processor and blend until smooth and creamy.

7. Transfer the soup back to the saucepan and season with sea salt and pepper.

8. Serve topped with yogurt and herbs.

ON THE SIDE: Turkey Breast and Mango Sandwich with Avocado (page 70)

PREP TIP: If you have a handheld immersion blender, use it to purée the soup right in the saucepan for one less dish to wash.

Per Serving: Calories: 241; Fat: 14g; Protein: 12g; Total Carbs: 15g; Fiber: 7g; Sodium: 121mg

CABBAGE-SALSA SOUP

Gluten-Free • Dairy-Free • Nut-Free

SERVES 4

PREP: 8 minutes

COOK: 22 minutes

1 tablespoon olive oil

1 sweet onion, chopped

2 celery stalks, diced

2 teaspoons minced garlic

4 cups shredded cabbage

2 carrots, diced

1 jalapeño pepper, seeded and finely chopped

1 (15-ounce) can sodium-free diced tomatoes

1 (15-ounce) can sodium-free navy beans

8 cups sodium-free chicken broth

Sea salt

Freshly ground black pepper

2 tablespoons chopped fresh cilantro

Cabbage soup may sound odd, but the complex taste and pleasing appearance of this dish will come as a welcome surprise. Plain green cabbage works best for color and texture, but you can use red or Napa varieties if they are already in your refrigerator. The leftover cabbage, about half a head, can be used in salads, juices, or as side dishes for other meals.

1. Place a large saucepan over medium-high heat and add the olive oil.

2. Sauté the sweet onion, celery, and garlic until the vegetables are tender, about 3 minutes.

3. Add the cabbage, carrots, and jalapeño pepper and sauté for 4 minutes.

4. Stir in the tomatoes, navy beans, and chicken broth.

5. Bring the soup to a boil, then reduce the heat to low and simmer until the vegetables are tender, about 15 minutes.

6. Season with sea salt and pepper.

7. Serve topped with the cilantro.

ON THE SIDE: A fresh green salad

SUBSTITUTION TIP: A bag of precut coleslaw mix will save a bit of preparation time and taste the same. Use this mixture in place of the cabbage and carrots, about 6 cups total.

Per Serving: Calories: 299; Fat: 7g; Protein: 20g; Total Carbs: 40g; Fiber: 14g; Sodium: 105mg

RAS EL HANOUT VEGETABLE SOUP

Gluten-Free • Nut-Free • Vegetarian

SERVES 4

PREP: 15 minutes

COOK: 30 minutes

1 tablespoon olive oil

1 sweet onion, chopped

2 celery stalks, chopped

1 tablespoon minced garlic

4 cups sodium-free vegetable broth

1 (15-ounce) can sodium-free diced tomatoes, undrained

1 (15-ounce) can sodium-free garbanzo beans, drained and rinsed

2 carrots, cut in half lengthwise and sliced into half rounds

1 potato, diced

1 red bell pepper, chopped

2 tablespoons *ras el hanout* spice mix

2 cups shredded kale

¼ cup plain yogurt, for garnish

My first visit to a spice market in Tripoli was life-changing as a chef; the scents could be enjoyed blocks away and the selection was staggering. The owner of a tiny shop handed me a blend called "head of the shop," or *ras el hanout*, and described the dozens of spices that made up the heady concoction. This blend is now available in most grocery stores in North America and is the base of this hearty soup. *Ras el hanout* is also a brilliant spice blend for meat, poultry, and vegetables.

1. Place a large stockpot over medium-high heat and add the olive oil.

2. Sauté the sweet onion, celery, and garlic until softened, about 3 minutes.

3. Stir in the vegetable broth, tomatoes, garbanzo beans, carrots, potato, red bell pepper, and *ras el hanout*.

4. Bring the soup to a boil, then reduce the heat to low and simmer until the vegetables are tender, about 20 minutes.

5. Stir in the kale during the last 5 minutes of cooking.

6. Serve topped with yogurt.

ON THE SIDE: Cucumber sticks, to help with the heat

LEFTOVERS TIP: If you can make this soup the day before you plan to serve it, the flavors will have a chance to mellow and deepen.

Per Serving: Calories: 397; Fat: 6g; Protein: 12g; Total Carbs: 68g; Fiber: 20g; Sodium: 68mg

CLASSIC BLACK BEAN SOUP

Gluten-Free • Nut-Free • Kids Love It

SERVES 4

PREP: 10 minutes

COOK: 20 minutes

1 tablespoon olive oil

1 sweet onion, chopped

1 tablespoon minced garlic

6 cups sodium-free chicken broth

2 (15-ounce) cans sodium-free black beans

1 teaspoon ground cumin

½ teaspoon ground coriander

Sea salt

Freshly ground black pepper

¼ cup prepared tomato salsa, for garnish

¼ cup sour cream, for garnish

1 tablespoon chopped fresh cilantro, for garnish

Some soups seem to be appropriate for specific seasons, such as gazpacho in the summer and asparagus soup in the spring. Black bean soup works year-round because it is hearty without being heavy, and the spices and colorful toppings make it look very fresh. If you go with dried beans instead of using canned, pick through them first to remove any stray rocks and debris.

1. Place a large stockpot over medium-high heat and add the olive oil.

2. Sauté the sweet onion and garlic until softened, about 3 minutes.

3. Add the chicken broth, black beans, cumin, and coriander and bring the soup to a boil.

4. Reduce the heat to low and simmer until the beans are tender, about 15 minutes.

5. Transfer the soup to a food processor or blender and purée until it is smooth and creamy.

6. Season the soup with sea salt and pepper.

7. Serve topped with salsa, sour cream, and cilantro.

ON THE SIDE: Avocado Chopped Salad (page 47)

VARIATION TIP: Add vegetables such as diced carrots, potatoes, and celery to the soup and do not purée it smooth. You can still top it with the salsa and sour cream.

Per Serving: Calories: 221; Fat: 6g; Protein: 16g; Total Carbs: 26g; Fiber: 10g Sodium: 70mg

CREAMY TOMATO SOUP

Gluten-Free • Nut-Free • Kids Love It

SERVES 4

PREP: 5 minutes

COOK: 20 minutes

1 tablespoon olive oil

1 sweet onion, chopped

2 celery stalks, chopped

1 tablespoon minced garlic

1 (28-ounce) can sodium-free crushed tomatoes

3 cups sodium-free chicken broth

¼ cup sodium-free tomato paste

1 tablespoon chopped fresh basil

1 teaspoon chopped fresh oregano

Sea salt

Freshly ground black pepper

½ cup plain yogurt

Chopped herbs (basil, chives, oregano), for garnish

The most requested lunch in my house when my kids were little featured creamy tomato soup and fresh-baked multigrain bread. We also enjoyed this combination with a fresh green salad for dinner. This recipe has a complex flavor from the fresh herbs and the tang of yogurt, but children will still ask for seconds. Tomatoes get more nutritious when cooked because heating this fruit increases the amount of lycopene, the phytonutrient that makes tomatoes red.

1. Place a large saucepan over medium-high heat and add the olive oil.

2. Sauté the sweet onion, celery, and garlic until the vegetables are tender, about 3 minutes.

3. Stir in the tomatoes, chicken broth, tomato paste, basil, and oregano.

4. Bring the soup to a boil and then reduce the heat to low and simmer for 15 minutes.

5. Purée the soup until very smooth in a food processor or with an immersion hand blender.

6. Season the soup with sea salt and pepper.

7. Serve topped with yogurt and herbs.

ON THE SIDE: Quinoa Salad–Stuffed Pita (page 69)

VARIATION TIP: Add chopped cooked chicken or turkey to the soup for a more substantial meal. You will not have to increase the cooking time with this additional ingredient.

Per Serving: Calories: 169; Fat: 5g; Protein: 8g; Total Carbs: 25g; Fiber: 8g; Sodium: 153mg

CHICKEN, KALE, AND PESTO SOUP

Gluten-Free • Kids Love It

SERVES 4

PREP: 7 minutes

COOK: 23 minutes

1 tablespoon olive oil

1 sweet onion, chopped

2 teaspoons minced garlic

8 cups sodium-free chicken broth

1 (15-ounce) can sodium-free great northern beans, drained and rinsed

2 cups chopped cooked chicken breast

2 celery stalks, chopped

2 carrots, diced

2 parsnips, diced

1 potato, peeled and diced

2 cups shredded kale

3 tablespoons basil pesto

Sea salt

Freshly ground black pepper

Centuries of home-remedy wisdom tout chicken soup as a cure for the sniffles, and regardless of the validity of these claims, there is no denying that this soup is comforting. Whip up a batch for a quick, filling meal on cold winter nights. If you plan on doubling the recipe for freezing, leave out the kale because it does not reheat well. Stir in the kale when reheating the soup so it stays vibrant and green.

1. Place a large stockpot over medium-high heat and add the olive oil.

2. Sauté the sweet onion and garlic until softened, about 3 minutes.

3. Stir in the chicken broth, great northern beans, chicken, celery, carrots, parsnips, and potato. Bring the soup to a boil, and then reduce the heat to low and simmer until the vegetables are tender, about 20 minutes.

4. In the last 5 minutes of cooking, stir in the kale and pesto.

5. Season with sea salt and pepper.

6. Serve.

ON THE SIDE: Mixed green salad

SUBSTITUTION TIP: If you have a favorite pesto recipe, you can use that instead of store-bought. Pesto is a staple item in clean eating because it can be used to enhance many types of recipes.

Per Serving: Calories: 437; Fat: 15g; Protein: 31g; Total Carbs: 45g; Fiber: 12g; Sodium: 197mg

QUINOA SALAD–STUFFED PITA

Dairy-Free • Nut-Free • Vegan • Vegetarian

SERVES 4

PREP: 20 minutes

COOK: 0 minutes

3 tablespoons olive oil

Juice of 1 lemon

1 teaspoon minced garlic

2 cups cooked quinoa

1 tomato, diced

1 yellow bell pepper, diced

½ English cucumber, diced

1 scallion, white and green parts, finely chopped

¼ cup finely chopped parsley

Sea salt

Freshly ground black pepper

4 whole-wheat pitas

1 cup shredded lettuce

As with most wraps and sandwiches, you can use almost any combination of ingredients to customize to your taste. This version is filling and fresh-tasting, but slices of cooked salmon or chicken breast would certainly make a delicious addition. Try a dollop of plain yogurt as a topping to give a Greek flair to your dinner.

1. In a large bowl, whisk together the olive oil, lemon, and garlic until blended.

2. Stir in the quinoa, tomato, yellow bell pepper, cucumber, scallion, and parsley.

3. Season the quinoa mixture with sea salt and pepper.

4. Cut the pitas in half and open them.

5. Spoon the quinoa mixture, divided evenly, into the pita halves and top with the shredded lettuce.

6. Serve.

ON THE SIDE: *Ras el Hanout* Vegetable Soup (page 65)

LEFTOVERS TIP: The quinoa salad used for the pitas is delicious on its own as a side or a snack, so double up on the recipe and store in the refrigerator in a sealed container for up to three days.

Per Serving: Calories: 398; Fat: 14g; Protein: 11g; Total Carbs: 61g; Fiber: 10g; Sodium: 378mg

TURKEY BREAST AND MANGO SANDWICH WITH AVOCADO

Dairy-Free • Nut-Free • Kids Love It

SERVES 4

PREP: 15 minutes

COOK: 0 minutes

1 avocado, peeled, pitted, and mashed

½ red bell pepper, finely chopped

1 tablespoon chopped cilantro

1 tablespoon freshly squeezed lemon juice

8 slices multigrain or whole-wheat bread

12 ounces cooked turkey breast, sliced

Sea salt

Freshly ground black pepper

1 mango, peeled, pitted, and sliced into strips

1 cup baby kale

Turkey, pale-green avocado, and bright mango look so stunning together that you might be tempted to just admire this sandwich instead of eating it. Mango is packed with antioxidants such as beta-carotene in addition to calcium, iron, amino acids, and vitamins A, C, and E. Try this bright fruit in savory and sweet dishes to help safeguard your health.

1. In a small bowl, stir together the avocado, red bell pepper, cilantro, and lemon juice until well mixed.

2. Place 4 bread slices on a clean work surface and spread the avocado mixture on the bread, dividing it evenly.

3. Top the avocado mixture with turkey slices and season it lightly with sea salt and pepper.

4. Top each slice with some mango, some kale, and the remaining 4 bread slices.

5. Serve.

ON THE SIDE: Creamy Tomato Soup (page 67)

VARIATION TIP: Whole-wheat tortillas can be used instead of bread as long as you eat the wrap right away. The juices from the avocado mixture and fresh mango can make the thin tortillas soggy if you wait too long.

Per Serving: Calories: 397; Fat: 12g; Protein: 24g; Total Carbs: 47g; Fiber: 10g; Sodium: 287mg

CHICKEN AND SUN-DRIED TOMATO WRAPS

Nut-Free

SERVES 4

PREP: 15 minutes

COOK: 0 minutes

2 ounces goat cheese

¼ cup chopped sun-dried tomatoes

2 teaspoons chopped fresh parsley

4 (8-inch) whole-wheat tortillas

16 ounces shredded cooked chicken breast

1 large ripe tomato, chopped

1 cup shredded spinach

For more than two decades, I lived in Wellington County in Southern Ontario, a location famous for the production of delicious goat cheese. Goat cheese forms the base of the creamy spread used on this sandwich. I often use this tangy cheese (one of my favorites) to enhance dinners in our house because it is nutritious and lactose-free. Use any extra goat cheese for sauces, soups, and salads.

1. In a small bowl, stir together the goat cheese, sun-dried tomatoes, and parsley until well mixed.

2. Place the tortillas on a clean work surface and spread each with the goat-cheese mixture.

3. Top with the chicken breast, tomatoes, and spinach.

4. Roll up the wraps and serve.

ON THE SIDE: Mixed green salad

PREP TIP: You will use chicken breasts quite frequently when eating clean, so prepping them in advance can save you time. Bake or poach 5 or 6 chicken breasts at the beginning of the week and store them in a sealed container in the refrigerator for up to 4 days, after cooling completely.

Per Serving: Calories: 294; Fat: 12g; Protein: 31g; Total Carbs: 13g; Fiber: 2g; Sodium: 364mg

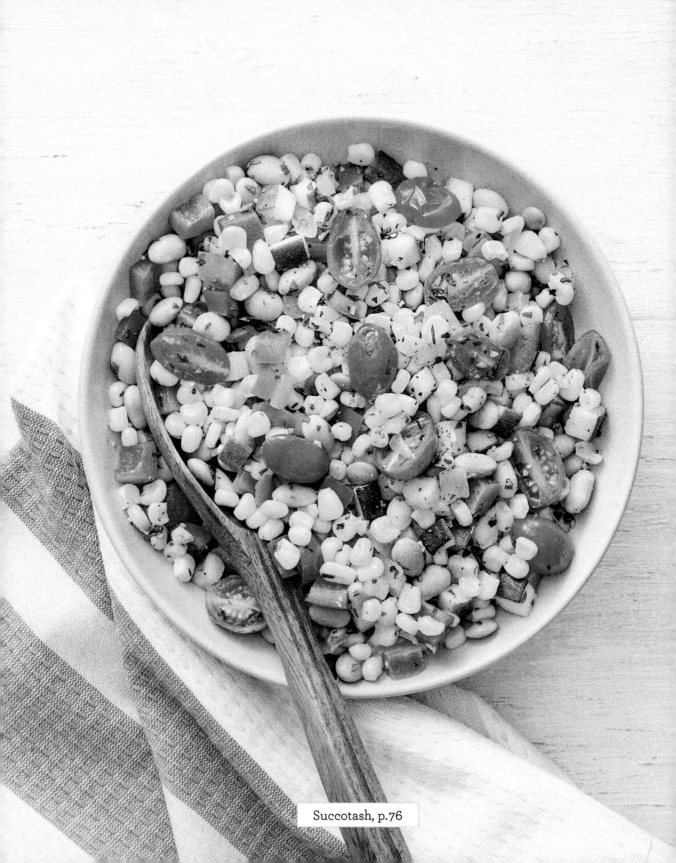

Succotash, p.76

6

SIDES

ROASTED SUMMER VEGETABLES

Gluten-Free • Dairy-Free • Nut-Free • Vegan • Vegetarian • Kids Love It

SERVES 4

PREP: 10 minutes

COOK: 30 minutes

2 tablespoons olive oil, divided

2 parsnips, cut into 1-inch chunks

1 carrot, cut into 1-inch chunks

1 sweet potato, cut into 1-inch chunks

¼ fennel bulb, sliced

1 cup halved fingerling potatoes

1 teaspoon fresh rosemary

4 beets, peeled and quartered

Sea salt

Freshly ground black pepper

Tender and lightly caramelized, roasted vegetables are a delight. As root vegetables cook, their flavor deepens and gets sweeter, especially carrots and sweet potatoes. Depending on your preference, you can also mash the finished vegetables with a little chicken or vegetable broth and top them with chopped almonds.

1. Preheat the oven to 400°F.
2. Line a baking sheet with parchment paper and set aside.
3. Toss 1½ tablespoons of the olive oil, parsnips, carrot, sweet potato, fennel, fingerling potatoes, and rosemary until well coated.
4. Spread the vegetable mixture over two-thirds of the baking tray.
5. Place the beets in the bowl with the remaining olive oil and toss to coat.
6. Spread the beets on the remaining one-third of the baking sheet.
7. Lightly season the vegetables with sea salt and pepper.
8. Roast the vegetables until tender and lightly browned, about 30 minutes.
9. Transfer the vegetables to a serving dish and serve.

LEFTOVERS TIP: Roasted vegetables are slightly sweet and are a welcome addition to smoothies, sauces, stews, and soups. You can add them whole to smoothies and any other recipe that is puréed, but you should chop them for other dishes.

Per Serving: Calories: 221; Fat: 7g; Protein: 4g; Total Carbs: 36g; Fiber: 8g; Sodium: 173mg

SUCCOTASH

Gluten-Free • Dairy-Free • Nut-Free • Vegan • Vegetarian

SERVES 8

PREP: 10 minutes
COOK: 15 minutes

1 tablespoon olive oil

½ sweet onion, chopped

1 teaspoon minced garlic

24 ounces cherry tomatoes, halved

2 cups corn kernels

1 cup shelled edamame

1 red bell pepper, diced

1 zucchini, diced

1 tablespoon apple cider vinegar

2 tablespoons chopped fresh parsley

1 tablespoon chopped fresh oregano

Freshly ground black pepper

Succotash is a traditional Southern dish made with corn, beans, tomatoes, and bell peppers. This inexpensive creation is a great choice to stay on budget or save a little money on your grocery bill. Add a little okra to the mixture if this vegetable is available in your area.

1. Place a large skillet over medium heat and add the olive oil.

2. Sauté the sweet onion and garlic until softened, about 3 minutes.

3. Add the tomatoes, corn, edamame, red bell pepper, and zucchini and cook for about 10 minutes, stirring occasionally, until the vegetables and edamame are heated through and tender.

4. Stir in the vinegar, parsley, and oregano.

5. Season with the pepper and serve.

LEFTOVERS TIP: This recipe makes a large quantity, which can be 4 heaping portions or 8 smaller ones, alongside an entrée. The leftovers can be served alone over brown rice or whole-wheat pasta for lunch the next day.

Per Serving: Calories: 190; Fat: 6g; Protein: 9g; Total Carbs: 29g; Fiber: 6g; Sodium: 34mg

LEMON-PEPPER SAUTÉED MUSHROOMS

Gluten-Free • Dairy-Free • Nut-Free • Vegan • Vegetarian • Kids Love It

SERVES 4

PREP: 10 minutes

COOK: 10 minutes

1 tablespoon olive oil

2 pounds button mushrooms, halved

1 teaspoon minced garlic

1 tablespoon freshly squeezed lemon juice

Sea salt

Freshly ground black pepper

Mushrooms combine well with grilled meats, poultry, and game meats as well as vegetarian entrées. Mushrooms are a wonderful source of iron, antioxidants, B vitamins, and vitamin D—they are the only vegetable source of this nutrient. Including them regularly in your meals can help boost your immune system and promote a healthy metabolism.

1. Place a large skillet over medium-high heat and add the olive oil.

2. Sauté the mushrooms, stirring frequently, until they are browned and tender, about 8 minutes.

3. Add the garlic and sauté for 2 minutes.

4. Remove the skillet from the heat, stir in the lemon juice and toss to coat.

5. Season the mushrooms with sea salt and pepper before serving.

PREP TIP: You can roast the mushrooms in a 350°F oven after tossing them with the oil and garlic. Bake them for 20 minutes and then transfer them to a serving bowl to stir in the lemon juice, sea salt, and pepper.

Per Serving: Calories: 81; Fat: 4g; Protein: 7g; Total Carbs: 8g; Fiber: 2g; Sodium: 72mg

GARLICKY OVEN-BAKED ZUCCHINI

Gluten-Free • Nut-Free • Vegetarian • Kids Love It

SERVES 4

PREP: 10 minutes

COOK: 15 minutes

2 teaspoons olive oil, plus more for the baking sheet

4 zucchini, cut into ½-inch slices

1 teaspoon minced garlic

2 tablespoons grated Parmesan cheese

Freshly ground black pepper

1 teaspoon chopped fresh parsley

Zucchini has an interesting, porous texture that was a little strange to me when I was young. My mother grew baskets of this vegetable and she threw it into baked goods, pasta, and soups on a daily basis at the end of the summer. When I tasted this cheesy, garlic-spiked recipe, I was sold on this vegetable for the rest of my life.

1. Preheat the oven to 400°F.

2. Lightly grease a baking sheet with olive oil.

3. In a medium bowl, toss together the olive oil, zucchini, and garlic until well coated.

4. Arrange the zucchini on the baking sheet in a single layer and sprinkle with the Parmesan cheese.

5. Bake until the zucchini is lightly caramelized and tender, about 15 minutes.

6. Season with pepper and top with parsley.

7. Serve.

LEFTOVERS TIP: Add the leftover cooked zucchini to pasta sauces, stews, or soups for extra flavor and texture.

Per Serving: Calories: 64; Fat: 3g; Protein: 4g; Total Carbs: 7g; Fiber: 2g; Sodium: 52mg

PUMPKIN WITH THYME

Gluten-Free • Dairy-Free • Nut-Free • Vegan • Vegetarian

SERVES 4

PREP: 10 minutes

COOK: 20 minutes

1½ pounds pumpkin, peeled, seeded, and cut into 1-inch chunks

1 tablespoon olive oil

1 tablespoon chopped fresh thyme

⅛ teaspoon ground nutmeg

Sea salt

Freshly ground black pepper

Pumpkin is not just for pies and puddings; this vibrant ingredient is also stellar for savory dishes. Pumpkin is very high in beta-carotene, potassium, vitamin A, and fiber, so it can help protect against cancer and heart disease. Look for smaller pie pumpkins because the flesh cooks up firm and it is the variety available at most grocery stores.

1. Preheat the oven to 450°F.

2. In a large bowl, toss the pumpkin, olive oil, thyme, and nutmeg until well coated.

3. Spread the pumpkin mixture on a baking sheet and season it lightly with sea salt and pepper.

4. Bake, stirring once, until the pumpkin is tender and lightly browned, about 20 minutes.

5. Serve.

SUBSTITUTION TIP: Fresh pumpkin is sometimes difficult to find in the grocery store, but good-quality frozen pumpkin is a perfectly acceptable substitute. Make sure you thaw the product before tossing it in the oil or the cooking time will be extended by about 25 minutes.

Per Serving: Calories: 92; Fat: 4g; Protein: 2g; Total Carbs: 16g; Fiber: 2g; Sodium: 61mg

MASHED SWEET POTATOES WITH APPLE

Gluten-Free • Nut-Free • Vegetarian • Kids Love It

SERVES 4

PREP: 10 minutes

COOK: 20 minutes

3 sweet potatoes, peeled and diced into large chunks

1 apple, peeled, cored, and diced

¼ cup plain yogurt

1 tablespoon maple syrup

½ teaspoon ground ginger

¼ teaspoon ground cinnamon

¼ teaspoon ground nutmeg

Sea salt

Freshly ground black pepper

Sweet potatoes are a staple in our kitchen; my kids adore the sweet flavor and pretty golden color. I like the fact that this vegetable provides a nutritional boost to my meals—and that I never have leftovers. A pear can be substituted for the apple in this recipe, just eliminate the maple syrup because pears tend to be a little sweeter.

1. Place the sweet potatoes and apple in a large saucepan and add water until the sweet potatoes and apple have 3 inches of water on top of them.

2. Bring the mixture to a boil over high heat and then reduce the heat to low and simmer until the vegetables are tender, about 20 minutes.

3. Drain the water and mash the potatoes and apple with the yogurt, maple syrup, ginger, cinnamon, and nutmeg until creamy.

4. Season with sea salt and pepper.

5. Serve.

LEFTOVERS TIP: If you have a few tablespoons of this side dish left after dinner, save it in a sealed container to use in a tasty smoothie the next day. Add it to any smoothie to add sweetness and a little rosy color.

Per Serving: Calories: 139; Fat: 0g; Protein: 3g; Total Carbs: 32g; Fiber: 5g; Sodium: 84mg

PARSNIP-CELERIAC PURÉE

Gluten-Free • Nut-Free • Vegetarian • Kids Love It

SERVES 4

PREP: 10 minutes

COOK: 15 minutes

2 parsnips, peeled and cut into 1-inch pieces

1 celeriac, peeled and cut into 1-inch pieces

½ cup plain yogurt

1 tablespoon maple syrup

½ teaspoon nutmeg

Sea salt

Mashed potatoes are often the first choice when considering this type of side dish, but other root vegetables have incredible texture and taste fabulous. Parsnip and celeriac create a creamy purée with a unique, earthy flavor. If you need a dairy-free version of this dish, use almond milk instead of yogurt in the same amount.

1. In a large saucepan, put the parsnip and celeriac in enough cold water to cover the vegetables.

2. Bring the water to a boil over high heat, and then reduce the heat to low.

3. Simmer until the vegetables are tender, about 10 to 15 minutes.

4. Drain and mash the vegetables with the yogurt, maple syrup, and nutmeg until smooth.

5. Season with sea salt and serve.

SUBSTITUTION TIP: This versatile recipe can also feature carrots, sweet potatoes, squash, or pumpkin. Use the same amounts of your new vegetable choice.

Per Serving: Calories: 152; Fat: 1g; Protein: 5g; Total Carbs: 32g; Fiber: 6g; Sodium: 194mg

CREAMED SPINACH AND KALE

Gluten-Free • Dairy-Free • Vegan • Vegetarian

SERVES 4

PREP: 7 minutes

COOK: 15 minutes

1 tablespoon olive oil

½ sweet onion, thinly sliced

2½ cups baby spinach, thoroughly washed

1 cup coarsely chopped kale, stemmed and thoroughly washed

½ cup vegetable broth

¼ cup coconut milk

¼ teaspoon ground nutmeg

Pinch sea salt

Pinch freshly ground black pepper

If you are not a fan of creamed vegetables, try this recipe before making up your mind completely. This dish is often overcooked, which creates a mushy texture and strange, pale-green sauce. The trick is to braise the greens until they are just wilted so they retain their integrity and the color does not leach out into the coconut-milk sauce.

1. Place a large skillet over medium heat and add the olive oil.

2. Add the sweet onion and sauté until lightly caramelized, about 5 minutes.

3. Stir in the baby spinach, kale, vegetable broth, coconut milk, nutmeg, sea salt, and pepper.

4. Cook, stirring occasionally, until the greens are wilted and the sauce is thickened, about 10 minutes.

5. Serve immediately.

SUBSTITUTION TIP: Frozen spinach or kale can be added if it is thawed first and all the excess liquid is squeezed out. Use the same amounts as the fresh greens.

Per Serving: Calories: 97; Fat: 6g; Protein: 3g; Total Carbs: 7g; Fiber: 3g; Sodium: 131mg

GOLDEN CORN PUDDING

Dairy-Free • Vegetarian • Kids Love It

SERVES 4

PREP: 10 minutes

COOK: 35 minutes

¾ cup unsweetened coconut milk, at room temperature

3 eggs

3 tablespoons coconut oil, melted, plus extra for greasing the baking pan

2 tablespoons honey

2 tablespoons whole-wheat flour

1 teaspoon baking powder

¼ teaspoon sea salt

4½ cups corn kernels

Fresh corn right off the cob is juicy and bursting with sweet flavor. When I was a child, my mother always told us to make a wish on the year's first fresh corn on the cob. I was always tempted to wish there was more corn on the table! Corn pudding was a familiar dish in my house and the recipe we used was adopted from our Pennsylvania Dutch relatives living in the States. If you have time, cut the corn kernels off the cob for a real treat.

1. Preheat the oven to 350°F.

2. Lightly grease an 8-by-8-inch square baking dish with coconut oil and set aside.

3. In a large bowl, stir together the coconut milk, eggs, coconut oil, and honey.

4. Stir together the flour, baking powder, and sea salt in a small bowl.

5. Add the dry ingredients to the wet ingredients and stir until smooth.

6. Stir the corn kernels into the batter until well mixed.

7. Spoon the batter into the baking dish and bake until the pudding is set, about 35 minutes.

8. Let the pudding cool for about 10 minutes. Serve warm.

SUBSTITUTION TIP: There are many high-quality flash-frozen vegetable products that are perfectly fine for clean-eating recipes. Try frozen corn kernels in the same amount after thawing them completely.

Per Serving: Calories: 314; Fat: 13g; Protein: 10g; Total Carbs: 45g; Fiber: 5g; Sodium: 188mg

BAKED TOMATO CASSEROLE

Dairy-Free • Nut-Free • Vegan • Vegetarian

SERVES 4

PREP: 10 minutes

COOK: 30 minutes

1 tablespoon olive oil, plus extra for greasing the casserole dish

2 slices whole-wheat or multigrain bread, cut into 1-inch cubes

2¼ pounds tomatoes, diced

2 teaspoons minced garlic

½ teaspoon freshly ground black pepper

3 tablespoons chopped fresh basil

1 tablespoon chopped fresh oregano

Bread puddings are usually thought to be sweet concoctions with chocolate and rich custard, but savory versions are popular, too. You will not find custard in this dish, but the tomatoes break down beautifully in the oven and soak into the bread chunks. Any type of tomato can be used, such as cherry tomatoes, plum, or beefsteak.

1. Preheat the oven to 350°F.

2. Lightly coat an 8-by-8-inch casserole dish with olive oil and set aside.

3. Place a large skillet over medium-high heat and add the olive oil.

4. Add the bread cubes and sauté until they're golden and crispy, about 3 minutes.

5. Add the tomatoes, garlic, and pepper and sauté for another 2 minutes.

6. Stir in the basil and oregano.

7. Transfer the tomato mixture to the casserole dish and bake until bubbly and browned, about 25 minutes.

8. Let the casserole cool for 10 minutes before serving.

LEFTOVERS TIP: Reheat the leftover casserole covered in the oven for 20 minutes and serve for breakfast topped with a poached or fried egg.

Per Serving: Calories: 178; Fat: 5g; Protein: 7g; Total Carbs: 30g; Fiber: 9g; Sodium: 84mg

BLACK BEAN PICO DE GALLO PILAF

Gluten-Free • Nut-Free • Vegetarian

SERVES 4

PREP: 15 minutes

COOK: 15 minutes

1 tablespoon olive oil

½ sweet onion, finely chopped

1 teaspoon minced garlic

1 teaspoon ground cumin

1 teaspoon ground coriander

1 (15-ounce) can sodium-free black beans

1 tomato, chopped

1 red bell pepper, chopped

1 jalapeño pepper, seeded and finely chopped

1 tablespoon chopped fresh cilantro

¼ cup low-sodium feta cheese, crumbled

Pico de gallo is an uncooked salsa made with tomatoes and a touch of spice, whereas the salsa you purchase in jars is made with cooked tomatoes. This difference makes the pico de gallo burst with fresh flavors—and makes it more perishable. If you have access to heirloom tomatoes, use an assortment of colors for an exceptional presentation.

1. Place a medium saucepan over medium-high heat and add the olive oil.

2. Sauté the sweet onion, garlic, cumin, and coriander until the vegetables are tender, about 3 minutes.

3. Add the black beans and reduce the heat to low. Cook the beans, stirring occasionally, until heated through, about 12 minutes.

4. While the beans are heating, combine the tomatoes, red bell pepper, jalapeño pepper, and cilantro in a small bowl.

5. Remove the beans from the heat and stir in the tomato mixture.

6. Serve the beans topped with feta cheese.

LEFTOVERS TIP: Spoon the bean mixture into pitas or wraps with a little chicken or sliced steak for a hearty lunch or light dinner. The mixture will keep in a sealed container in the refrigerator for up to three days.

Per Serving: Calories: 126; Fat: 6g; Protein: 6g; Total Carbs: 14g; Fiber: 4g; Sodium: 108mg

TRADITIONAL BAKED BEANS
WITH COLLARD GREENS

Gluten-Free • Dairy-Free • Nut-Free • Vegan • Vegetarian • Kids Love It

SERVES 6

PREP: 5 minutes

COOK: 25 minutes

1 tablespoon olive oil

½ sweet onion, chopped

2 teaspoons minced garlic

1 (15-ounce) can sodium-free crushed tomatoes

1 (15-ounce) can sodium-free pinto beans, drained and rinsed

1 (15-ounce) can sodium-free navy beans, drained and rinsed

2 tablespoons maple syrup

Sea salt

2 cups chopped collard greens

Navy beans get their name from their popularity as an ingredient enjoyed by the sailors in the US Navy. Baked beans with greens is a classic preparation, especially in the American South. You can use dried beans or canned beans in this recipe, but if you go with dried, increase the cooking time by at least 1 hour.

1. Place a large saucepan over medium-high heat, add the olive oil, and sauté the sweet onion and garlic until softened, about 3 minutes.

2. Stir in the tomatoes, pinto beans, navy beans, and maple syrup.

3. Bring the mixture to just below boiling and then reduce the heat to low and simmer until the beans are very tender, about 15 minutes.

4. Use a potato masher to mash about ¼ of the beans and stir them into the rest.

5. Season the beans with sea salt.

6. Stir in the collard greens and simmer until wilted, about 5 minutes.

7. Serve.

PREP TIP: If you have a little extra time, bake the beans in a 350°F oven in a covered casserole dish until very tender, about 45 minutes total. Add ¼ cup of water to the ingredients to avoid a dry result.

Per Serving: Calories: 241; Fat: 3g; Protein: 12g; Total Carbs: 42g; Fiber: 12g; Sodium: 46mg

WILD MUSHROOM–HAZELNUT RICE

Gluten-Free • Dairy-Free • Vegan • Vegetarian

SERVES 4

PREP: 4 minutes

COOK: 26 minutes

1 tablespoon olive oil

1½ cups sliced wild mushrooms

½ sweet onion, chopped

2 teaspoons minced garlic

1 cup uncooked brown basmati rice

2 cups sodium-free vegetable broth

Freshly ground black pepper

½ cup chopped hazelnuts

1 tablespoon chopped fresh parsley

If you have the time, spread the hazelnuts on a baking sheet and bake them in a 300°F oven until toasted and very fragrant. Let them cool slightly and rub the skins off the nuts. This extra step creates a decadent, rich flavor, especially when combined with earthy wild mushrooms.

1. Place a large saucepan over medium-high heat and add the olive oil.

2. Add the mushrooms, sweet onion, and garlic and sauté until lightly caramelized, about 5 minutes.

3. Stir in the rice and sauté an additional minute.

4. Add the vegetable broth and bring the mixture to a boil.

5. Reduce the heat to low and simmer, covered, until the liquid is absorbed and the rice is tender, about 20 minutes.

6. Season with pepper.

7. Top the rice with the hazelnuts and parsley.

8. Serve.

VARIATION TIP: Any type of grain such as bulgur, quinoa, or wheat berries can be used instead of rice in the same amount. Make sure you rinse the quinoa well to remove the soapy coating called saponins before adding it to the saucepan.

Per Serving: Calories: 152; Fat: 9g; Protein: 5g; Total Carbs: 14g; Fiber: 3g; Sodium: 15mg

WHOLE-GRAIN PENNE WITH SPINACH PESTO

Vegetarian • Kids Love It

SERVES 4

PREP: 10 minutes

COOK: 20 minutes

FOR THE PESTO

¼ cup spinach leaves

2 tablespoons fresh basil leaves

2 tablespoons fresh oregano leaves

2 tablespoons pine nuts

1 tablespoon grated Asiago cheese

1 teaspoon minced garlic

2 tablespoons olive oil

Freshly ground black pepper

FOR THE PENNE

4 ounces dry whole-grain penne

1 cup halved cherry tomatoes

½ cup chopped artichoke hearts

Pesto is one of those condiments that can be made with almost any ingredient, from herbs to dark leafy greens to sun-dried tomatoes. This variation highlights the deep, almost grassy flavor of spinach with a hint of fresh basil. If you like a lighter-tasting pasta, use less pesto, adding it by tablespoons until you arrive at your desired result.

TO MAKE THE PESTO

1. In a blender or food processor, pulse the spinach, basil, oregano, pine nuts, Asiago cheese, and garlic until very finely chopped.

2. Add the olive oil and pulse until a thick paste forms, about 2 minutes. Scoop the pesto into a bowl and set aside.

TO MAKE THE PENNE

1. Fill a large pot with water and bring it to a boil over high heat.

2. When the water is boiling, cook the pasta al dente, according to package directions.

3. Drain the pasta and return it to the pot. Stir in the pesto, tomatoes, and artichoke hearts.

4. Toss to combine and heat for 5 minutes.

5. Serve immediately.

LEFTOVERS TIP: Double up on the pesto recipe and store the extra in the refrigerator for up to one week to use as a tempting spread or as flavoring for soups and stews.

Per Serving: Calories: 220; Fat: 11g; Protein: 7g; Total Carbs: 24g; Fiber: 5g; Sodium: 34mg

SAVORY OATMEAL RISOTTO

Gluten-Free • Vegetarian

SERVES 8

PREP: 10 minutes

COOK: 25 minutes

1 tablespoon olive oil, plus extra for greasing the baking dish

1 sweet onion, chopped

2 teaspoons minced garlic

1 red bell pepper, chopped

1 cup chopped kale

2½ cups unsweetened almond milk

1 egg

2 cups large-flake old-fashioned oats

1 teaspoon chopped fresh thyme

1 teaspoon baking powder

¼ cup grated Parmesan cheese

Oatmeal might seem like an unusual ingredient for a savory side dish but it tastes similar to basmati rice and is gluten-free. Do not use quick oats for this dish or you will end up with a gluey mess rather than a pleasing texture. Try toasting the oats before adding them to the skillet for a toasty, rich flavor.

1. Preheat the oven to 350°F.

2. Lightly grease an 8-by-11-inch baking dish with olive oil and set aside.

3. Place a large skillet over medium-high heat and add the olive oil.

4. Add the sweet onion and garlic and sauté until tender, about 3 minutes.

5. Stir in the red bell pepper and kale and sauté for 2 minutes more.

6. Remove the skillet from the heat and stir in the almond milk, egg, oats, thyme, and baking powder until well mixed.

7. Transfer the oat mixture to the baking dish and sprinkle the top with Parmesan cheese.

8. Bake until the oats are tender and liquid is absorbed, about 20 minutes.

9. Serve.

PREP TIP: The entire recipe can be prepared ahead and stored in the refrigerator, covered with plastic wrap, until you are ready to make dinner. Remove the covering and pop the dish in a 350°F oven and bake for about 30 minutes.

Per Serving: Calories: 181; Fat: 9g; Protein: 6g; Total Carbs: 20g; Fiber: 4g; Sodium: 103mg

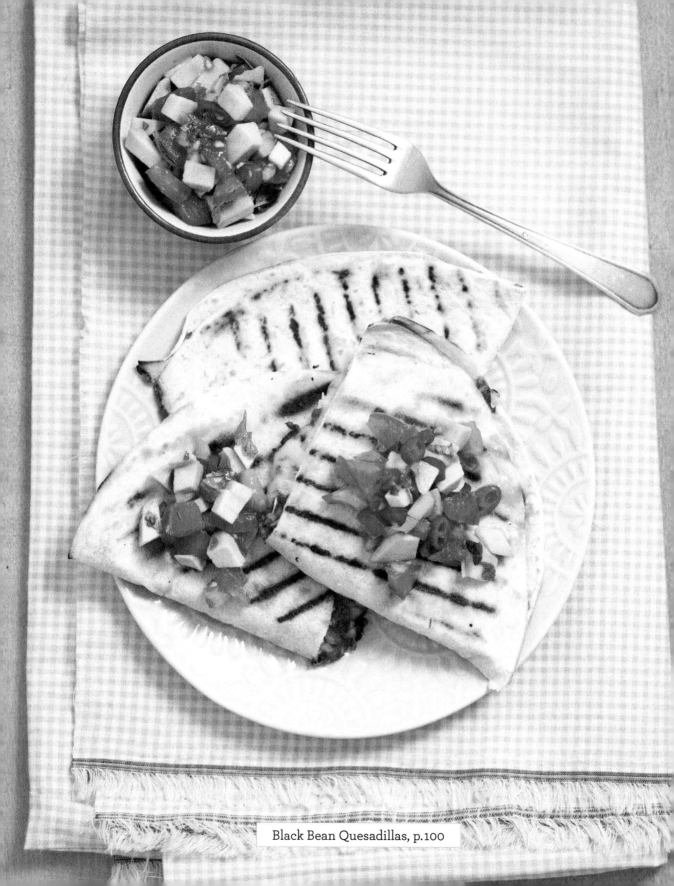

Black Bean Quesadillas, p.100

7

VEGETARIAN

SPICY CASHEW TOFU

Gluten-Free • Dairy-Free • Vegan • Vegetarian

SERVES 4

PREP: 10 minutes

COOK: 20 minutes

2 tablespoons sesame oil

2 tablespoons grated
fresh ginger

1 tablespoon minced garlic

1 (14-ounce) package extra-
firm tofu, drained and cut
into 1-inch cubes

1 red bell pepper,
thinly sliced

1 yellow bell pepper,
thinly sliced

2 scallions, white and green
parts, sliced thinly on a bias

1½ cups quartered bok choy

3 tablespoons tamari

2 tablespoons rice vinegar

Pinch red pepper flakes

¼ cup chopped cashews

Tofu can be an acquired taste, and I hid this ingredient in recipes for years so my family would eat it. They've come to appreciate the way that tofu soaks up the flavors of the dish, and they enjoy the lightly crispy texture when it is sautéed. The chopped cashews add a delightful crunch and richness to this dish. Cashews are considered to be tree nuts but they are the seeds from the cashew apple. Cashews, which are lower in fats than other nuts, are a stellar source of heart-healthy monounsaturated oleic acid.

1. Place a large skillet or wok over high heat and add the sesame oil.

2. Sauté the ginger and garlic for 2 minutes.

3. Add the tofu and sauté it until it is golden, about 5 minutes.

4. Add the red and yellow bell peppers, scallions, and bok choy and sauté until the vegetables are tender, about 5 to 6 minutes.

5. Stir in the tamari, rice vinegar, and red pepper flakes and toss to coat.

6. Serve immediately, topped with the chopped cashews.

ON THE SIDE: Brown basmati rice

VARIATION TIP: The vegetables can be changed depending on your personal preference or what you have in your refrigerator. Try snow peas, sliced carrots, broccoli florets, or bean sprouts for an interesting variation.

Per Serving: Calories: 463; Fat: 22g; Protein: 38g; Total Carbs: 27g; Fiber: 8g; Sodium: 460mg

QUINOA-STUFFED ACORN SQUASH

Gluten-Free • Dairy-Free • Vegan • Vegetarian • Kids Love It

SERVES 4

PREP: 10 minutes

COOK: 30 minutes

FOR THE SQUASH

2 acorn squash, cut in half, seeds scooped out

1 teaspoon olive oil

The only time I had a serious injury during my decades of cooking happened because an acorn squash rolled when I tried to cut it in half. After that incident, I always pop this squash in the microwave for about 30 seconds to soften the skin slightly before cutting. This compact squash is the perfect size to fill with grains, meats, vegetables, and dried fruit for a substantial meal.

To save time, you can roast the squash several days in advance and store it, seeded and halved, in the refrigerator in a sealed container. Let the squash come to room temperature, fill, and bake for 20 minutes in a 350°F oven.

TO MAKE THE SQUASH

1. Preheat the oven to 350°F.

2. Line a baking sheet with parchment paper.

3. Lightly oil the cut sides of the squash with olive oil and place them cut-side down on the baking sheet.

4. Bake the squash until tender, about 30 minutes.

5. Remove the squash from the oven and flip it over.

6. Scoop out a couple tablespoons of flesh from each half to make the hollow deeper. (This extra squash can be added to the prepared filling, if desired.)

FOR THE FILLING

1 tablespoon olive oil

¾ sweet onion,
finely chopped

1 celery stalk, chopped

1 teaspoon
minced garlic

1 cup shredded kale

2 cups cooked quinoa

½ cup dried cranberries

¼ cup chopped
hazelnuts

1 teaspoon chopped
fresh thyme

Sea salt

Freshly ground
black pepper

TO MAKE THE FILLING

1. While the squash is cooking, place a large skillet over medium heat and add the olive oil.

2. Sauté the sweet onion, celery, and garlic until softened, about 4 minutes.

3. Stir in the kale and sauté until wilted, about 4 minutes.

4. Remove the skillet from the heat and stir in the reserved squash (if desired), quinoa, dried cranberries, hazelnuts, and thyme.

5. Season the filling with sea salt and pepper.

6. Spoon the filling evenly into the cooked squash halves.

7. Serve warm.

PREP TIP: The entire recipe can be prepared ahead of time and popped in the oven directly from the refrigerator when you get home from work. Bake the stuffed squash until heated through, about 30 minutes.

Per Serving: Calories: 286; Fat: 9g; Protein: 8g; Total Carbs: 47g; Fiber: 8g; Sodium: 81mg

VEGETABLE-LENTIL FRITTATA

Gluten-Free • Dairy-Free • Nut-Free • Vegetarian

SERVES 4

PREP: 10 minutes

COOK: 20 minutes

1 tablespoon olive oil

¼ sweet onion, chopped

2 teaspoons minced garlic

1 zucchini, diced

1 cup asparagus, cut into 1-inch pieces

½ yellow bell pepper, diced

1 cup shredded Swiss chard

1 cup halved cherry tomatoes

8 large eggs, beaten

1 cup cooked red lentils

Sea salt

Freshly ground black pepper

I love packing a staggering amount of colorful vegetables into this golden frittata: dark leafy greens, tomatoes, vibrant peppers, and bright-green asparagus. When lentils are added to the combination, you have a filling meal on the table in a mere 30 minutes! Garnish the frittata with sprigs of thyme or basil leaves for a fresh finishing touch.

1. Preheat the oven to 425°F.

2. Place a large ovenproof skillet over medium-high heat and add the olive oil.

3. Sauté the sweet onion and garlic until softened, about 3 minutes.

4. Stir in the zucchini, asparagus, yellow bell pepper, Swiss chard, and cherry tomatoes and sauté until the vegetables are tender, about 5 minutes.

5. In a medium bowl, whisk together the eggs and lentils.

6. Pour the eggs into the skillet.

7. Cook the frittata until the eggs are almost cooked through and set, lifting the edges to let the raw egg flow underneath, about 10 minutes.

8. Place the skillet in the preheated oven. Bake the frittata until the top is set, about 5 minutes.

9. Remove the frittata from the oven and let it stand for 5 minutes.

10. Season with salt and pepper, cut into quarters, and serve.

ON THE SIDE: Mixed green salad

VARIATION TIP: This frittata is also delicious with whole-grain penne instead of the lentils, which adds more texture and substance. Cook the pasta and cool it completely before adding it to the eggs.

Per Serving: Calories: 266; Fat: 12g; Protein: 21g; Total Carbs: 18g; Fiber: 6g; Sodium: 257mg

WILD RICE BOWL

Gluten-Free • Vegetarian

SERVES 4

PREP: 15 minutes

COOK: 15 minutes

FOR THE DRESSING

3 tablespoons olive oil

Juice and zest of 1 lime

1 tablespoon honey

1 tablespoon chopped fresh cilantro

1 teaspoon fresh ginger, peeled and grated

FOR THE RICE BOWL

2 cups cooked wild rice

1 cup cooked quinoa

1 cup cooked garbanzo beans

1 cup thinly shredded kale

1 red bell pepper, thinly sliced

1 carrot, grated

½ cup dried cranberries

½ cup chopped hazelnuts

1 scallion, white and green parts, sliced thin on a bias

Bowls are a culinary trend taking home kitchens and fine-dining restaurants by storm. Bowls in this context are when lots of different ingredients are combined or layered in one bowl rather than spread out on a plate. This dinner choice includes grains, grasses, legumes, vegetables, nuts, and fruit tossed in a tart but sweet dressing. Delicious and satisfying!

TO MAKE THE DRESSING

1. In a small bowl, whisk together the olive oil, lime juice and zest, honey, cilantro, and ginger until blended.

2. Set aside.

TO MAKE THE RICE BOWL

1. In a large bowl, toss together the wild rice, quinoa, garbanzo beans, kale, red bell pepper, carrot, cranberries, and hazelnuts until well mixed.

2. Add the dressing and stir to combine.

3. Serve topped with the scallion.

PREP TIP: This recipe tastes even better the next day because the flavors mellow, so make the entire dish the day before you want to serve it.

Per Serving: Calories: 396; Fat: 16g; Protein: 13g; Total Carbs: 50g; Fiber: 10g; Sodium: 48mg

MUSHROOM FRIED BROWN RICE

Gluten-Free • Dairy-Free • Nut-Free • Vegetarian

SERVES 4

PREP: 7 minutes

COOK: 23 minutes

2 tablespoons olive oil

½ sweet onion, chopped

2 teaspoons minced garlic

1 teaspoon grated
fresh ginger

4 cups sliced mushrooms

4 cups cooked brown
basmati rice

2 tablespoons chopped
fresh cilantro

2 tablespoons tamari

2 eggs, beaten

1 scallion, white and
green parts, chopped

You can easily create a healthy version of Chinese fried rice at home with all the flavor of the restaurant dish. If you want a vegan version, leave out the scrambled eggs and add a little tofu instead. Cut the tofu into ½-inch cubes and sauté them along with the mushrooms.

1. Place a large skillet over medium-high heat and add the olive oil.

2. Sauté the sweet onion, garlic, and ginger until softened, about 3 minutes.

3. Stir in the mushrooms and sauté until lightly caramelized, about 7 minutes.

4. Add the rice, cilantro and tamari.

5. Sauté, stirring constantly, for about 10 minutes or until the rice is heated through.

6. Move the rice to the side of the skillet and pour in the eggs.

7. Scramble the eggs, for about 3 minutes total, and mix them into the rice.

8. Serve topped with the scallion.

ON THE SIDE: Garlicky Oven-Baked Zucchini (page 78)

VARIATION TIP: Although plain button mushrooms are delicious, try a combination of mushrooms for the very best results. Shiitake, oyster, enoki, and portobello are all wonderful choices.

Per Serving: Calories: 277; Fat: 11g; Protein: 10g; Total Carbs: 38g; Fiber: 4g; Sodium: 382mg

BLACK BEAN QUESADILLAS

Nut-Free • Vegetarian • Kids Love It

SERVES 4

PREP: 15 minutes

COOK: 15 minutes

Nonstick cooking spray

8 (6-inch) whole-wheat tortillas

2 (15-ounce) cans sodium-free black beans, drained and rinsed

1 red bell pepper, seeded and diced

1 jalapeño pepper, seeded and coarsely chopped

1 scallion, white and green parts, chopped

1 tablespoon chopped fresh cilantro

1 teaspoon ground cumin

1 tomato, diced

½ cup firm goat cheese, crumbled

Salsa, for garnish (optional)

Quesadillas are traditionally folded in half rather than layered as in this version. You can top this savory treat with corn, herbs, potato, pumpkin, or mushrooms depending on your personal taste. Set out an assortment of toppings and let your family create their own special quesadillas. You can serve these with a spoonful of avocado or tomato salsa.

1. Preheat the oven to 450°F.

2. Lightly coat 2 baking sheets with the cooking spray and place 2 tortillas on each sheet.

3. In a food processor, pulse the black beans, red bell pepper, jalapeño pepper, scallion, cilantro, and cumin until coarsely chopped.

4. Spread the bean mixture onto the tortillas on the baking sheet and then top them with the tomato and goat cheese.

5. Place the remaining 4 tortillas on top and bake them in the oven, turning once, until the tortillas are crispy and lightly browned and the filling is heated through and bubbly, about 15 minutes.

6. Cut the quesadillas into quarters, garnish with the salsa (if desired), and serve.

ON THE SIDE: Guacamole

PREP TIP: You can also use a barbecue set to medium heat to make the quesadillas. Simply prepare them and heat them through, turning once, about 6 minutes total.

Per Serving: Calories: 394; Fat: 11g; Protein: 26g; Total Carbs: 52g; Fiber: 22g; Sodium: 293mg

ZUCCHINI ENCHILADAS

Gluten-Free • Nut-Free • Vegetarian • Kids Love It

SERVES 4

PREP: 7 minutes

COOK: 23 minutes

4 zucchini, cut in half and scooped out, leaving ¼ inch of flesh

1 tablespoon olive oil

1 sweet onion, chopped

2 teaspoons minced garlic

2 (15-ounce) cans sodium-free black beans, drained and rinsed

2 tomatoes, chopped

1 red bell pepper, chopped

1 jalapeño pepper, seeded and chopped

2 teaspoons chili powder

1 teaspoon ground cumin

½ cup goat cheese

2 tablespoons chopped fresh cilantro

Enchiladas might not be an accurate description for these stuffed vegetables, but the filling is quite close and they are delicious. To increase the similarity to the real dish, you can drizzle enchilada sauce over the top of the filling before adding goat cheese. To save time, prepare the recipe beforehand and store it in the refrigerator until you get home from work, and then bake it until heated through and bubbly.

1. Preheat the oven to 400°F and line a baking sheet with parchment paper.

2. Arrange the zucchini cut-side up on the baking sheet.

3. Place a large skillet over medium-high heat and add the olive oil.

4. Sauté the sweet onion and garlic until softened, about 3 minutes.

5. Add the black beans, tomatoes, red bell pepper, jalapeño pepper, chili powder, and cumin and sauté for another 5 minutes.

6. Spoon the filling into the zucchini and top them with the goat cheese.

7. Bake the boats until the zucchini is tender, about 15 minutes.

8. Top with the cilantro and serve.

PREP TIP: Choose zucchini that are about 8 inches long and not too skinny, or there won't be enough room for the filling. Save the scooped-out zucchini flesh for smoothies, sauces, and soups.

Per Serving: Calories: 393; Fat: 10g; Protein: 24g; Total Carbs: 55g; Fiber: 20g; Sodium: 89mg

GARBANZO BEAN BURGERS

Dairy-Free • Nut-Free • Vegetarian • Kids Love It

SERVES 4

PREP: 15 minutes,
plus 1 hour chilling time

COOK: 10 minutes

2 cups cooked garbanzo
beans, rinsed and drained

½ cup cooked quinoa

¼ cup whole-wheat
bread crumbs

2 eggs

¼ cup grated carrots

1 scallion, white and green
parts, chopped

1 teaspoon minced garlic

1 teaspoon dried oregano

Pinch red pepper flakes

Pinch sea salt

1 tablespoon olive oil

Vegetable burgers have a long history of strange flavor profiles—either they have no taste or too strong of a taste (and sometimes both at the same time). But people now demand high-quality vegetarian choices as this style of eating has become more popular, so veggie burgers have since come a long way. These burgers look appetizing and have a slightly nutty flavor.

1. In a food processor, pulse the garbanzo beans, quinoa, bread crumbs, eggs, carrots, scallion, garlic, oregano, red pepper flakes, and sea salt until the mixture is well combined and holds together.

2. Press the mixture into 4 equal patties and place them, covered, in the refrigerator until firm, about 1 hour.

3. Place a large skillet over medium-high heat and add the olive oil.

4. Brown the patties on both sides and heat through, turning once, about 10 minutes.

5. Serve.

ON THE SIDE: Succotash (page 76)

VARIATION TIP: Serve the patties plain or on a multigrain bun with your favorite toppings. Try tomatoes, pickles, sliced onion, and a little pesto to create unique flavor combinations.

Per Serving: Calories: 486; Fat: 11g; Protein: 24g; Total Carbs: 68g; Fiber: 26g; Sodium: 150mg

ASPARAGUS-THYME FARFALLE

Nut-Free • Vegetarian • Kids Love It

SERVES 4

PREP: 10 minutes

COOK: 15 minutes

1 tablespoon olive oil

1 tablespoon minced garlic

1 cup sodium-free vegetable broth

Juice and zest of 1 lemon

4 cups cooked whole-wheat farfalle

2 cups asparagus spears, trimmed and cut into 2-inch pieces

¼ cup grated Parmesan cheese

I have a favorite pasta. I don't mean an exotic flavor such as squid ink or turmeric; I like farfalle pasta above all else. My preference for this jaunty little frilled bow tie has infected my kids and they'll ask specifically for farfalle even when the recipe calls for something else. The shape of farfalle looks very attractive with the bright asparagus spears in this recipe. Asparagus is high in vitamin A and is considered to be an antioxidant and anti-inflammatory.

1. Place a large skillet over medium-high heat and add the olive oil.

2. Sauté the garlic until softened, about 2 minutes.

3. Add the vegetable broth, lemon juice and zest, pasta, and asparagus and sauté, stirring constantly, until the pasta is heated through and the asparagus is tender, about 10 minutes.

4. Serve topped with Parmesan cheese.

ON THE SIDE: A tossed green salad

PREP TIP: Any type of pasta will keep in the refrigerator for up to five days when stored in a sealed container after it is cooled completely. Toss a teaspoon of olive oil with the pasta to prevent it from sticking together.

Per Serving: Calories: 282; Fat: 6g; Protein: 11g; Total Carbs: 45g; Fiber: 4g; Sodium: 68mg

SUN-DRIED TOMATO AND KALAMATA OLIVE LINGUINE

Vegetarian

SERVES 4

PREP: 15 minutes

COOK: 15 minutes

FOR THE PESTO

½ cup sun-dried tomatoes, packed in water

¼ cup fresh basil leaves

2 tablespoons pine nuts

2 garlic cloves

1 tablespoon olive oil

Freshly ground black pepper

FOR THE PASTA

8 ounces whole-wheat linguine

½ cup sliced Kalamata olives

1 cup torn spinach

Pinch red pepper flakes

¼ cup grated Parmesan cheese

Black olives are not all created equally, which is why you'll want to use Kalamata olives for this dish. Kalamatas are large, purplish-black olives picked when they are ripe for full flavor. They are a protected product under EU law, grown only near the town of Kalamata in Peloponnese Greece. The extra expense of these olives is well worth it.

TO MAKE THE PESTO

1. In a food processor or blender, pulse the sun-dried tomatoes, basil, pine nuts, garlic, and olive oil until a thick paste forms.

2. Season the pesto with pepper and set aside.

TO MAKE THE PASTA

1. While making the pesto, cook the linguine in boiling water according to package instructions.

2. Drain the pasta and toss it with the pesto, olives, spinach, and red pepper flakes until well coated.

3. Serve topped with Parmesan cheese.

ON THE SIDE: Mixed green salad

PREP TIP: The pesto can be made in advance and stored in the refrigerator in a sealed container for up to one week. If you have extra, spread it on sandwiches and stir into soups to add extra flavor.

Per Serving: Calories: 483; Fat: 13g; Protein: 22g; Total Carbs: 80g; Fiber: 12g; Sodium: 258mg

EGGPLANT-TOMATO TAGINE

Gluten-Free • Nut-Free • Vegan • Vegetarian

SERVES 4

PREP: 10 minutes

COOK: 1 hour and 30 minutes

Olive oil, for greasing the casserole dish

1 (28-ounce) can sodium-free diced tomatoes, undrained

½ cup low-sodium vegetable broth

2 eggplants, cubed

2 zucchini, diced

½ sweet onion, chopped

1 tablespoon minced garlic

1 teaspoon ground cumin

½ teaspoon ground coriander

¼ teaspoon ground turmeric

Pinch cayenne pepper powder

½ cup plain yogurt

2 tablespoons chopped fresh parsley

A tagine is a cone-shaped cooking pot used to create stews in North African cooking. I encountered this interesting vessel while working in Libya and Tunisia as a chef for several ambassadors. The design of the pot condenses every delectable drop of moisture released by the cooking ingredients back into the broth. The casserole dish and lid used for this spicy recipe work in a similar fashion.

1. Preheat the oven to 350°F.

2. Lightly grease a 2-quart casserole dish with the olive oil.

3. In the casserole dish, stir together the tomatoes, vegetable broth, eggplant, zucchini, sweet onion, garlic, cumin, coriander, turmeric, and cayenne pepper powder.

4. Cover and bake until the vegetables are very tender, about 1½ hours.

5. Serve topped with the plain yogurt and parsley.

ON THE SIDE: Serve with brown basmati rice or whole-wheat couscous

PREP TIP: If you have a slow cooker, this recipe can be made on low heat for 6 to 8 hours with no changes to the ingredient amounts.

Per Serving: Calories: 153; Fat: 1g; Protein: 8g; Total Carbs: 33g; Fiber: 13g; Sodium: 40mg

BUTTERNUT SQUASH
AND CANNELLINI STEW

Gluten-Free • Dairy-Free • Nut-Free • Vegan • Vegetarian

SERVES 4

PREP: 10 minutes

COOK: 20 minutes

1 tablespoon olive oil

1 sweet onion, chopped

1 tablespoon minced garlic

1 (28-ounce) can sodium-free diced tomatoes, undrained

4 cups diced butternut squash

1 (15-ounce) can sodium-free cannellini beans

2 parsnips, diced

1 cup sodium-free vegetable broth

1 tablespoon ground cumin

1 teaspoon chili powder

½ teaspoon cinnamon

2 cups baby spinach

Sea salt

Freshly ground black pepper

Squash is an inspired addition to stews because of its bright color and hint of sweetness. Squash is packed with antioxidants such as alpha-carotene, beta-carotene, lutein, and zeaxanthin, making it a potent disease fighter. Butternut squash is also an excellent source of vitamins A, B_6, and C, as well as fiber, manganese, and copper.

1. Place a large saucepan over medium-high heat and add the olive oil.

2. Sauté the sweet onion and garlic for about 3 minutes, or until softened.

3. Stir in the tomatoes, squash, cannellini beans, parsnips, vegetable broth, cumin, chili powder, and cinnamon.

4. Bring the mixture to a boil. Reduce the heat to low, and simmer until the vegetables are tender, about 15 to 17 minutes.

5. Stir in the spinach in the last 5 minutes of cooking time.

6. Season with sea salt and pepper.

7. Serve.

ON THE SIDE: Cooked quinoa or whole-grain couscous

PREP TIP: If you want to make this stew in a slow cooker, add the ingredients, cover, and cook on high heat for 3 to 4 hours or on low heat for 6 to 8 hours.

Per Serving: Calories: 260; Fat: 5g; Protein: 9g; Total Carbs: 50g; Fiber: 15g; Sodium: 126mg

LENTIL AND POTATO STEW

Gluten-Free • Dairy-Free • Nut-Free • Vegan • Vegetarian

SERVES 4

PREP: 7 minutes

COOK: 23 minutes

1 tablespoon olive oil

1 sweet onion,
finely chopped

2 teaspoons minced garlic

2 cups vegetable broth

1 (28-ounce) can sodium-free diced tomatoes,
undrained

2 (15-ounce) cans sodium-free lentils, drained

2 potatoes, peeled and
cut into 1-inch cubes

1 carrot, diced

1 teaspoon chopped
fresh thyme

1 teaspoon chopped
fresh oregano

Sea salt

Freshly ground
black pepper

A simple, hearty stew can be exactly what your family needs on days that seem too long and too busy. Sit down to a quiet meal and enjoy this herb-infused dinner with a nice salad or a comforting dessert. Try a dollop of plain yogurt or a sprinkle of feta cheese for a bit of extra protein.

1. Place a large saucepan over medium-high heat and add the olive oil.

2. Sauté the sweet onion and garlic until the vegetables are softened, about 3 minutes.

3. Stir in the vegetable broth, tomatoes, lentils, potatoes, carrot, thyme, and oregano and bring to a boil.

4. Reduce the heat to medium-low and simmer the stew until the vegetables are tender, about 20 minutes.

5. Season with sea salt and pepper.

6. Serve.

ON THE SIDE: Avocado Chopped Salad (page 47)

LEFTOVERS TIP: Leftover stew can be spooned into whole-wheat pitas or over brown basmati rice for a satisfying hot lunch. Reheat it in a small saucepan for about 10 minutes after removing from the refrigerator.

Per Serving: Calories: 367; Fat: 4g; Protein: 20g; Total Carbs: 60g; Fiber: 20g; Sodium: 157mg

KALE CASSOULET

Gluten-Free • Dairy-Free • Nut-Free • Vegan • Vegetarian • Kids Love It

SERVES 4

PREP: 10 minutes

COOK: 20 minutes

1 tablespoon olive oil

½ sweet onion, chopped

2 teaspoons minced garlic

4 cups chopped kale

2 cups cooked black beans

2 cups cooked garbanzo beans

2 cups cooked great northern beans

½ cup low-sodium vegetable broth

1 teaspoon ground smoked paprika

1 teaspoon ground cumin

1 teaspoon dried oregano

¼ teaspoon ground cayenne pepper powder

Sea salt

Freshly ground black pepper

1 tablespoon chopped fresh oregano

One-dish casseroles are a staple in my house because they are inexpensive, can be made in advance, and make for manageable cleanup when children are wrangled to do the dishes. *Cassoulet* is just a fancier French name for a bean-based casserole. Traditional *cassoulet* includes pork, but this vegetarian version has kale instead.

1. Place a large saucepan over medium-high heat and add the olive oil.

2. Sauté the sweet onion and garlic for about 3 minutes, or until softened.

3. Add the kale and sauté for 2 more minutes, or until wilted.

4. Stir in the black beans, garbanzo beans, great northern beans, vegetable broth, paprika, cumin, oregano, and cayenne pepper powder.

5. Bring the mixture to a boil. Reduce the heat to low, and simmer for 15 minutes. Remove from the heat, and season with sea salt and pepper.

6. Sprinkle with the oregano and serve.

LEFTOVERS TIP: For a tasty lunch, spoon the bean mixture over some brown rice or into a whole-grain pita. If you use it for sandwich filling, you do not have to heat it up beforehand.

Per Serving: Calories: 435; Fat: 6g; Protein: 23g; Total Carbs: 70g; Fiber: 25g; Sodium: 148mg

HEARTY VEGETABLE CHILI

Gluten-Free • Dairy-Free • Nut-Free • Vegan • Vegetarian • Kids Love It

MEAL PLAN
WEEK 2
FRIDAY

SERVES 4

PREP: 15 minutes

COOK: 30 minutes

1 tablespoon olive oil

1 sweet onion, chopped

2 teaspoons minced garlic

1 green bell pepper, diced

1 red bell pepper, diced

1 large zucchini, diced

1 jalapeño pepper, seeded and finely chopped

1 (28-ounce) can sodium-free diced tomatoes, undrained

1 (15-ounce) can sodium-free red kidney beans, drained

1 (15-ounce) can sodium-free navy beans, drained

3 tablespoons chili powder

1 tablespoon ground cumin

Pinch cayenne pepper powder

Chili is my go-to choice when I need a nutritious meal quickly with little effort. The combination of beans in this version packs both protein and fiber. You can make chili in a slow cooker if you want the meal ready when your family walks in the door. Set the slow cooker on low for 8 to 10 hours, or on high for 6 hours, depending on your schedule.

1. Place a large stockpot on medium-high heat and add the olive oil.

2. Sauté the sweet onion and garlic until softened, about 3 minutes.

3. Add the green bell pepper, red bell pepper, zucchini, and jalapeño pepper and sauté for 5 minutes.

4. Stir in the diced tomatoes, red kidney beans, navy beans, chili powder, cumin, and cayenne pepper powder.

5. Bring the chili to a boil and then reduce the heat to low.

6. Simmer until the flavors have mellowed, about 20 minutes.

7. Remove the chili from the heat and let it stand for about 10 minutes before serving.

ON THE SIDE: Golden Corn Pudding (page 83)

VARIATION TIP: Chili powder is the traditional flavoring for this dish, but chipotle chili powder adds a luscious smoky flavor that is unique and pleasing. Start with 2 tablespoons of the chipotle chili powder and add a little more if you want a more intense flavor.

Per Serving: Calories: 321; Fat: 6g; Protein: 17g; Total Carbs: 53g; Fiber: 18g; Sodium: 177mg

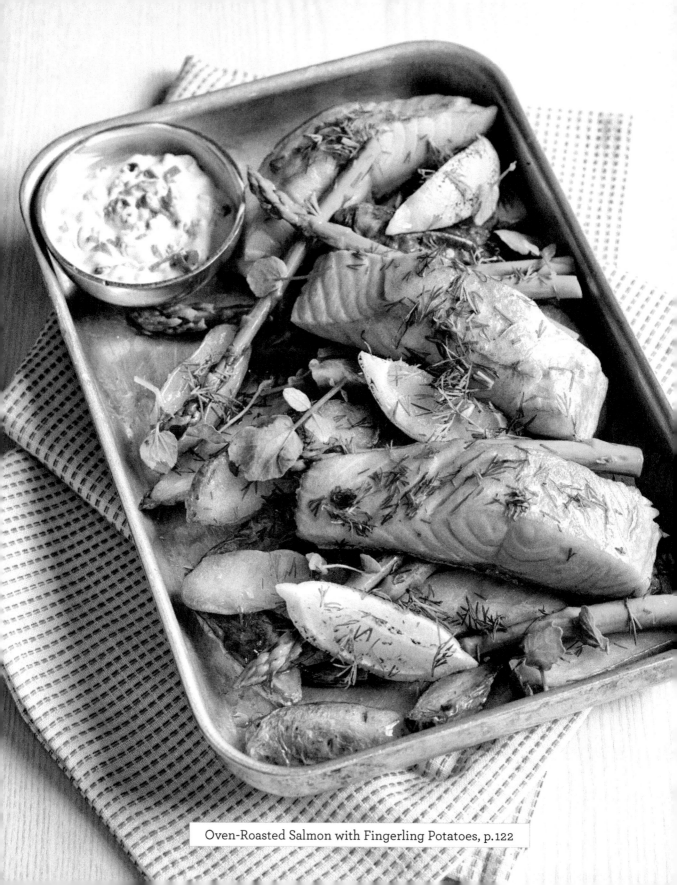

Oven-Roasted Salmon with Fingerling Potatoes, p.122

8

SEAFOOD

SEAFOOD-STUFFED AVOCADOS

Gluten-Free • Kids Love It

SERVES 4

PREP: 15 minutes

COOK: 0 minutes

2 avocados, pitted

¼ pound cooked shrimp, peeled, deveined, and chopped

¼ pound cooked crab meat

1 scallion, white and green parts, chopped

½ red bell pepper, finely chopped

½ carrot, grated

¼ cup plain yogurt

Juice of 1 lemon

Sea salt

Freshly ground black pepper

Fresh cilantro, for garnish

Although the portion size looks small, the avocado, vegetables, and seafood are surprisingly filling. Avocado is packed with the healthy fats and fiber that are hallmarks of clean eating. The outermost, dark-green portion of the pulp that you leave in this recipe has the highest concentration of phytonutrients, so dig in and enjoy.

1. Scoop out avocados, leaving a ½-inch thickness of fruit in each half. Chop the removed flesh and transfer it to a medium bowl.

2. Stir in the shrimp, crab, scallion, red bell pepper, carrot, yogurt, and lemon juice.

3. Season the mixture with sea salt and pepper.

4. Spoon the mixture into the avocado halves and top with the cilantro.

5. Serve.

ON THE SIDE: Black Bean Pico de Gallo Pilaf (page 85)

PREP TIP: If your avocados are not ripe enough, wrap them tightly in foil and place them in a 200°F oven for up to 10 minutes. Check the progress of the fruit after about 5 minutes.

Per Serving: Calories: 284; Fat: 20g; Protein: 13g; Total Carbs: 12g; Fiber: 7g; Sodium: 328mg

SEA SCALLOPS WITH COCONUT SAUCE

Gluten-Free • Dairy-Free • Nut-Free

SERVES 4

PREP: 10 minutes

COOK: 20 minutes

1 pound sea scallops, rinsed and patted dry

Sea salt

Freshly ground black pepper

1 tablespoon olive oil

½ sweet onion, finely chopped

1 red bell pepper, cut into thin strips

1 yellow bell pepper, cut into thin strips

1 scallion, white and green parts, chopped

1 cup light coconut milk

1 tablespoon red chili paste

1 teaspoon grated fresh ginger

2 tablespoons chopped fresh cilantro

People who don't like seafood often enjoy sea scallops because these mollusks are sweet and mild-tasting. Although scallops are available frozen year-round, look for them fresh from late fall to early spring. Scallops are extremely high in vitamin B_{12}, iodine, phosphorous, and protein.

1. Season the scallops with sea salt and pepper.

2. Heat the olive oil in a large skillet over medium-high heat.

3. Pan sear the scallops until they are browned and crisp on one side, about 3 minutes. Carefully turn them over and sear the other side until browned and crisp, about 3 minutes.

4. Transfer the seared scallops to a plate and cover them loosely with foil to keep them warm.

5. Return the skillet to medium heat and sauté the onion, red bell pepper, yellow bell pepper, and scallion until tender, about 5 minutes.

6. Stir in the coconut milk, red chili paste, and ginger and bring the sauce to a simmer, stirring, about 5 minutes.

7. Reduce the heat to low and return the scallops to the skillet.

8. Turn the scallops to coat them with the sauce.

9. Serve topped with cilantro.

ON THE SIDE: Roasted Summer Vegetables (page 75)

SUBSTITUTION TIP: Bay scallops are smaller and sweeter than sea scallops, so they will cook quicker if you want to try them in this recipe. Sometimes the smaller product is more readily available in supermarkets.

Per Serving: Calories: 311; Fat: 18g; Protein: 22g; Total Carbs: 15g; Fiber: 3g; Sodium: 248mg

SHRIMP WITH ROASTED PEPPERS AND FETA

Nut-Free • Kids Love It

SERVES 4

PREP: 10 minutes

COOK: 20 minutes

1 (28-ounce) can sodium-free diced tomatoes

1 cup diced roasted red peppers

½ red bell pepper, diced

1 tablespoon minced garlic

1 tablespoon chopped fresh basil

Pinch red pepper flakes

24 medium shrimp, peeled and deveined

2 tablespoons freshly squeezed lemon juice

½ cup low-sodium feta cheese, crumbled

8 ounces dried whole-grain spaghetti

Shrimp may not be your first choice for most dinners, but when you do serve it finding a simple recipe is invaluable. This complex-tasting sauce is created in the oven with little to no effort; all you have to do is cook the pasta—and relax. If you want to add more color to your meal, stir a cup of baby spinach or shredded kale into the simmering spaghetti just before the pasta is completely cooked.

1. Preheat the oven to 450°F.

2. In a 9-by-13-inch baking dish, toss together the tomatoes, roasted red peppers, red bell pepper, garlic, basil, and red pepper flakes.

3. Top with the shrimp, lemon juice, and feta cheese.

4. Bake until the shrimp are cooked through and the sauce is bubbly, about 20 minutes.

5. While the shrimp is baking, cook the spaghetti according to package instructions.

6. Serve the spaghetti topped with the sauce and shrimp.

ON THE SIDE: Mixed green salad

SUBSTITUTION TIP: You can peel and devein the shrimp yourself, but to save time, purchase precleaned product, either fresh or frozen. Thaw the frozen shrimp completely before using it in this dish.

Per Serving: Calories: 611; Fat: 5g; Protein: 81g; Total Carbs: 54g; Fiber: 6g; Sodium: 276mg

CRAB-STUFFED SOLE PARMESAN

Nut-Free • Kids Love It

SERVES 4

PREP: 10 minutes

COOK: 15 minutes

6 ounces lump crabmeat

¼ cup whole-wheat bread crumbs, divided

¼ cup grated Parmesan cheese

1 tablespoon chopped chives

1 teaspoon chopped dill

4 (6-ounce) sole fillets

Unless you live where crab is common, such as the Pacific Northwest, California, or Alaska, this shellfish feels decadent. Creating a stuffing of crabmeat allows you to get all the delicious goodness without great expense; look for good-quality canned or frozen products for the best results.

1. Preheat the oven to 350°F.

2. Line a baking sheet with parchment paper and set aside.

3. In a small bowl, stir together the crabmeat, 2 tablespoons of bread crumbs, Parmesan cheese, chives, and dill.

4. Pat the sole fillets dry with paper towels and place them on a clean work surface.

5. Spoon the crab mixture into the center of each fillet and roll the fillets around the filling to form cylinders. Place the rolled fish seam-side down in the baking dish.

6. Sprinkle the tops with the remaining bread crumbs.

7. Bake the fish until it is cooked through, about 15 minutes.

8. Serve immediately.

ON THE SIDE: Roasted Summer Vegetables (page 75)

SUBSTITUTION TIP: Frozen crabmeat is a delicious option as long as it is real and not the brightly colored imitation crab. Thaw the crab completely and squeeze out the extra moisture before adding it to the other ingredients.

Per Serving: Calories: 260; Fat: 7g; Protein: 50g; Total Carbs: 2g; Fiber: 0g; Sodium: 318mg

SPICY FISH STEW

Gluten-Free • Dairy-Free • Nut-Free

SERVES 4

PREP: 10 minutes

COOK: 30 minutes

1 tablespoon olive oil

1 sweet onion, chopped

2 celery stalks, diced

2 teaspoons minced garlic

1 (28-ounce) can sodium-free diced tomatoes

1 cup sodium-free chicken broth

2 carrots, diced

¼ fennel bulb, cut into thin strips

1 pound boneless, skinless fish, cut into 1-inch pieces

1 cup baby spinach

¼ teaspoon red pepper flakes

Sea salt

Freshly ground black pepper

1 tablespoon chopped fresh basil

Many names are used all around the world for describing fish stew; this dish crosses cultural and geographic lines easily. The closest to this version of stew is probably *cacciucco*, an Italian stew with Turkish origins. To create a more authentic stew, use several types of fish and add shrimp or mussels, too.

1. Place a large saucepan over medium-high heat and add the olive oil.

2. Sauté the sweet onion, celery, and garlic until softened, about 3 minutes.

3. Add the tomatoes, chicken broth, carrots, and fennel and bring to a boil.

4. Reduce the heat to low and simmer until the vegetables are tender, about 15 minutes.

5. Stir in the fish, spinach, and red pepper flakes and increase the heat to medium.

6. Simmer the stew until the fish is cooked through, about 10 minutes.

7. Season with sea salt and pepper.

8. Serve topped with the basil.

ON THE SIDE: Brown basmati rice

VARIATION TIP: Firm fish should be used for this stew because more-tender fish can break up when heated. For the best results, try salmon, halibut, haddock, or tilapia.

Per Serving: Calories: 171; Fat: 4g; Protein: 22g; Total Carbs: 12g; Fiber: 3g; Sodium: 285mg

SHORE-LUNCH TROUT

Gluten-Free • Dairy-Free • Nut-Free

SERVES 4

PREP: 5 minutes

COOK: 8 minutes

4 (6-ounce) trout fillets, skinned

Sea salt

Freshly ground black pepper

Sweet paprika, for seasoning

2 tablespoons olive oil

2 teaspoons chopped fresh dill

1 lemon, cut into 8 wedges

My home now is in Northern Ontario, Canada, where lakes are around every corner of the road. Bass, walleye, perch, and lake trout are easily obtainable as long as you have a good fishing rod and a couple of hours to spend on the water. The method of cooking this recipe might seem excessively simple, but it allows the sweet, firm flesh of the fish to shine through. You can cook cut-up fingerling potatoes and sliced sweet onion in the same skillet as the fish for a true shore-lunch experience.

1. Wash the fish fillets, pat dry with paper towels, and season with salt, pepper, and paprika.

2. Place a large skillet over medium-high heat and add the olive oil.

3. Pan sear the fish for 4 minutes on each side, or until just cooked through and golden brown.

4. Sprinkle the fish with dill and serve with lemon wedges.

ON THE SIDE: Wild Mushroom–Hazelnut Rice (page 87)

SUBSTITUTION TIP: Fresh-caught fish is the best choice for this recipe, but you can get very nice trout in many supermarkets.

Per Serving: Calories: 181; Fat: 12g; Protein: 17g; Total Carbs: 0g; Fiber: 0g; Sodium: 89mg

CHILI-LIME CATFISH

Gluten-Free • Dairy-Free • Nut-Free • Kids Love It

SERVES 4

PREP: 10 minutes

COOK: 12 minutes

4 (6-ounce) catfish fillets

1 teaspoon chili powder

½ teaspoon garlic powder

¼ teaspoon cayenne
pepper powder

1 tablespoon olive oil

Juice of 1 lime

Chopped cilantro,
for garnish

Lime wedges, for garnish

Catfish is often left off healthy diets because it is associated with deep-fried dishes in southern United States. As with many ingredients, preparation is the key to creating a nutritious meal. Baking this fish results in a low-calorie, high-protein meal, which is rich in omega-3 fatty acids, selenium, and vitamin B_{12}. For the freshest fish, look for those that have a mild or neutral odor and firm flesh.

1. Preheat the oven to 400°F. Line a baking sheet with foil and set aside.

2. Pat the catfish fillets dry with paper towels and place them on the baking sheet. Set aside.

3. In a small bowl, stir together the chili powder, garlic powder, and cayenne pepper powder.

4. Rub the spice mixture into the fish, on both sides, and place the fillets back on the baking tray.

5. Sprinkle the olive oil and lime juice over the fish and bake until the catfish flakes, about 12 minutes.

6. Serve topped with the cilantro and lime wedges.

ON THE SIDE: Black Bean Pico de Gallo Pilaf (page 85)

VARIATION TIP: Any white fish can be used in this simple recipe, such as tilapia, sole, halibut, or haddock. Adjust the cooking time depending on the thickness of the fillet.

Per Serving: Calories: 263; Fat: 16g; Protein: 26g; Total Carbs: 1g; Fiber: 0g; Sodium: 97mg

HALIBUT TACOS WITH AVOCADO SALSA

Nut-Free • Kids Love It

SERVES 4

PREP: 15 minutes

COOK: 10 minutes

FOR THE SALSA

1 avocado, peeled, pitted, and diced

1 tomato, chopped

1 scallion, white and green parts, chopped

2 tablespoons chopped cilantro

2 tablespoons freshly squeezed lime juice

Sea salt

Freshly ground black pepper

FOR THE TACOS

1 tablespoon olive oil

4 (4-ounce) halibut fillets

Sea salt

Freshly ground black pepper

4 (6-inch) whole-grain tortillas

Halibut is a mild-tasting, firm fish with an almost buttery-smooth texture when cooked perfectly. If you are concerned with sustainably caught fish, look for halibut from the Pacific waters off British Columbia, Alaska, and California. Before serving these tacos, let the salsa come to room temperature because the taste of the avocado will be stronger.

TO MAKE THE SALSA

1. In a small bowl, stir together the avocado, tomato, scallion, cilantro, and lime juice.

2. Season with sea salt and pepper.

3. Set aside.

TO MAKE THE TACOS

1. Place a large skillet over medium-high heat and add the olive oil.

2. Pat the halibut dry with paper towels and season with sea salt and pepper.

3. Pan fry the fish until cooked through and the halibut flakes easily with a fork, turning once, about 10 minutes.

4. Arrange the tortillas on a clean work surface.

5. Place a fish fillet in the middle of each tortilla. Spoon the salsa on the fish and fold the tortillas in half.

6. Serve.

ON THE SIDE: Succotash (page 76)

LEFTOVERS TIP: The avocado salsa is delicious as a topping for chicken, sandwiches, and soup. It can also be used with baked pita chips as a lovely snack. Store the salsa in the refrigerator in a sealed container for up to three days.

Per Serving: Calories: 510; Fat: 19g; Protein: 63g; Total Carbs: 16g; Fiber: 5g; Sodium: 314mg

SALMON BURGERS WITH JICAMA SLAW

Nut-Free • Kids Love It

SERVES 4

PREP: 15 minutes

COOK: 10 minutes

FOR THE SLAW

1 jicama, peeled and grated

1 carrot, grated

1 parsnip, grated

1 scallion, white and green parts, chopped

1 tablespoon freshly squeezed lemon juice

1 tablespoon honey

2 tablespoons chopped fresh cilantro leaves

FOR THE BURGERS

16 ounces cooked salmon

½ cup whole-wheat bread crumbs

2 eggs

1 scallion, white and green parts, chopped

¼ red bell pepper, finely chopped

2 tablespoons plain yogurt

1 tablespoon prepared horseradish

⅛ teaspoon salt

Freshly ground black pepper

2 tablespoons olive oil

4 whole-grain buns

When I was young, every few weeks we had "fish day," which meant a plate of cardboard-textured fish sticks served with lots of ketchup. Instead of prepackaged fish sticks, my children experienced fresh-made moist salmon burgers, sans ketchup. Since the salmon in this recipe is cooked, you can either use leftovers from another meal or good-quality canned salmon packed in broth. Oil-packed salmon adds unwanted oil to the burgers.

TO MAKE THE SLAW

In a medium bowl, toss together the jicama, carrot, parsnip, scallion, lemon juice, honey, and cilantro. Set aside.

TO MAKE THE BURGERS

1. In a medium bowl, stir together the salmon, bread crumbs, eggs, scallion, red bell pepper, yogurt, horseradish, salt, and pepper until the mixture holds together when pressed.

2. Shape the mixture into 4 patties.

3. Place a large skillet over medium heat and add the olive oil.

4. Cook the burgers until browned, turning once, about 5 minutes per side.

5. Serve on buns with a generous scoop of jicama slaw.

ON THE SIDE: Black Bean Pico de Gallo Pilaf (page 85)

PREP TIP: Put together the burgers and wrap each burger individually in plastic wrap. Store the burgers in the freezer for up to one month and thaw them in the refrigerator overnight when you wish to cook them.

Per Serving: Calories: 398; Fat: 10g; Protein: 32g; Total Carbs: 48g; Fiber: 16g; Sodium: 356mg

OVEN-ROASTED SALMON WITH FINGERLING POTATOES

Gluten-Free · Dairy-Free · Nut-Free · Kids Love It

SERVES 4

PREP: 10 minutes

COOK: 20 minutes

2 tablespoons olive oil, divided, plus extra to grease the baking dish

4 (5-ounce) salmon fillets

Sea salt

Freshly ground black pepper

1 pound blanched fingerling potatoes, halved

12 asparagus spears, trimmed

2 teaspoons minced garlic

1 tablespoon freshly squeezed lemon juice

2 tablespoons chopped chives

1 tablespoon chopped dill

Lemon wedges, for garnish

Fresh herbs, for garnish

Cleaning salmon was one of the tests I needed to pass to work with one of the best chefs in Southern Ontario. When I say cleaning salmon, I mean whole salmon— I had to cut the fillets off the carcass, skin, debone, and cut the fillets into perfect 6-ounce portions. There were 25 of them, so I learned to really appreciate this gorgeous, firm fish. Baking salmon with vegetables makes for a wonderful one-dish dinner.

1. Preheat the oven to 400°F.

2. Lightly grease a 9-by-13-inch baking dish with olive oil.

3. Pat the fish dry with paper towels and season with sea salt and pepper. Set aside.

4. In a large bowl, toss together the fingerling potatoes, asparagus, garlic, and 1½ tablespoons of the olive oil.

5. Spread the vegetables in the baking dish and top with the salmon fillets.

6. Drizzle the remaining ½ tablespoon of the olive oil on the fish along with the lemon juice.

7. Sprinkle the chives and dill on the vegetables and fish.

8. Bake until the fish is cooked through and the vegetables are tender, about 17 to 20 minutes.

9. Serve with lemon wedges topped with fresh herbs.

ON THE SIDE: Whole-Grain Penne with Spinach Pesto (page 88)

SUBSTITUTION TIP: This cooking technique is very effective for any type of seafood, including shrimp and scallops. Vary the vegetables and herbs depending on what is in season.

Per Serving: Calories: 272; Fat: 8g; Protein: 38g; Total Carbs: 12g; Fiber: 4g; Sodium: 119mg

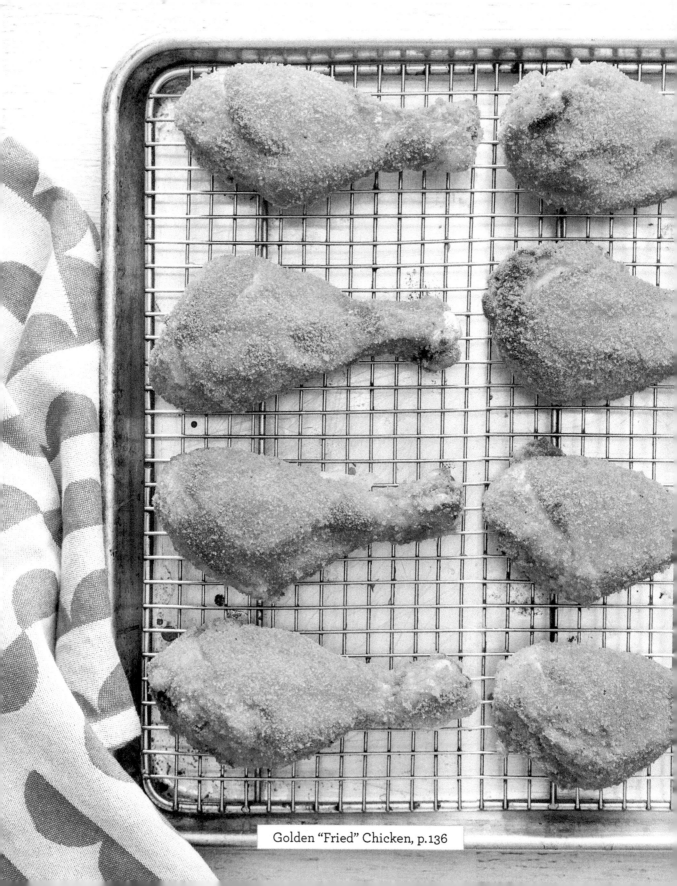

Golden "Fried" Chicken, p.136

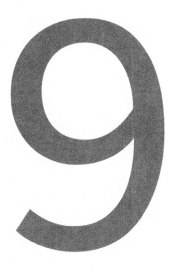

9

POULTRY

TURKEY-COUSCOUS SKILLET

Dairy-Free • Nut-Free • Kids Love It

SERVES 4

PREP: 10 minutes

COOK: 20 minutes

1 tablespoon olive oil

1 sweet onion, chopped

2 teaspoons minced garlic

2 celery stalks, chopped

1 parsnip, grated

1 carrot, grated

1 cup green beans, trimmed and cut into 1-inch pieces

1 cup chopped cauliflower

2 cups chopped cooked turkey

2 cups cooked Israeli couscous

2 teaspoons chopped fresh basil

Turkey is not only for Thanksgiving; this tasty bird can be included in your weekly meal plans as a healthy choice in casseroles and soups. If possible, get organic and pasture-raised turkey; it has more healthy omega-3 content than conventionally farmed birds. Turkey can help lower post-meal insulin levels, as only 4 ounces of the meat contain 35 grams of protein and less than 1 gram of fat.

1. Preheat the oven to 400°F.

2. Place a large ovenproof skillet over medium-high heat and add the olive oil.

3. Sauté the sweet onion, garlic, celery, parsnip, carrot, green beans, and cauliflower until softened, about 10 minutes.

4. Stir in the turkey, couscous, and basil.

5. Place the skillet in the oven, covered, and bake until the turkey and couscous are heated through, about 10 minutes.

6. Serve.

ON THE SIDE: Mashed Sweet Potatoes with Apple (page 80)

SUBSTITUTION TIP: Israeli couscous is larger than regular couscous so it remains firm and holds its shape when baked in the oven. But you can certainly use regular couscous if you don't mind a dish with a little less texture.

Per Serving: Calories: 299; Fat: 7g; Protein: 26g; Total Carbs: 32g; Fiber: 6g; Sodium: 82mg

TURKEY-KALE ENCHILADAS

Gluten-Free • Nut-Free • Kids Love It

SERVES 4

PREP: 10 minutes

COOK: 20 minutes

1 tablespoon olive oil, plus extra for greasing the baking dish

1 cup low-sodium enchilada sauce, divided

½ sweet onion, chopped

1 jalapeño pepper, seeded and chopped

1 teaspoon chili powder

1 teaspoon ground cumin

1 pound boneless, skinless turkey breasts, cooked and chopped

1 (15-ounce) can sodium-free white beans, drained and rinsed

8 large kale leaves, hard ribs cut out

½ cup goat cheese, divided

2 tablespoons chopped fresh cilantro

Kale leaves replace the traditional tortillas in this dish, creating a delectable gluten-free version. Select an enchilada sauce with very little sodium or make your own. The jalapeño pepper adds a hot element to the dish because this vegetable contains a substance called capsaicin. Capsaicin is used medicinally for boosting immunity, for weight loss, and for reducing the pain associated with psoriasis and arthritis.

1. Preheat the oven to 400°F.

2. Lightly grease an 8-by-8-inch baking dish with olive oil and spread ¼ cup of the enchilada sauce on the bottom.

3. Place a large skillet over medium-high heat and add the olive oil.

4. Sauté the sweet onion, jalapeño pepper, chili powder, and cumin until the vegetables are softened, about 3 minutes.

5. Stir in the turkey and white beans, and sauté 5 minutes more.

6. Lay a kale leaf on a cutting board and spoon about ¼ cup of the filling in the center.

7. Top with the goat cheese and fold the sides of the leaf over the filling. Then roll the leaf to form a tight packet.

8. Place the roll in the baking dish and repeat with the remaining ingredients.

9. Pour the remaining sauce over the rolls and bake until the leaves are tender, about 10 minutes.

10. Serve topped with the fresh cilantro.

ON THE SIDE: Golden Corn Pudding (page 83)

VARIATION TIP: Try ground beef or chicken instead of turkey if that suits your palate better. This dish can also be made with whole-wheat tortillas instead of kale if you want a more substantial meal.

Per Serving: Calories: 469; Fat: 15g; Protein: 54g; Total Carbs: 26g; Fiber: 8g; Sodium: 217mg

HONEY DIJON CHICKEN
WITH SHAVED VEGETABLE SALSA

Gluten-Free • Dairy-Free • Nut-Free • Kids Love It

SERVES 4

PREP: 15 minutes

COOK: 30 minutes

FOR THE CHICKEN

1 tablespoon olive oil

4 (4-ounce) boneless, skinless chicken breasts

¼ cup honey

3 tablespoons Dijon mustard

1 teaspoon sweet paprika

1 teaspoon dried thyme

FOR THE SALSA

¼ fennel bulb, grated

2 yellow beets, peeled and grated

1 carrot, grated

1 apple, cored and grated

1 tablespoon freshly squeezed lemon juice

1 tablespoon honey

Sea salt

Freshly ground black pepper

Dijon is a prepared mustard from the city of Dijon, in the Burgundy region of France. White wine, spices, and brown mustard seeds create its distinct flavor. Do not substitute other types of mustard because they won't give you the same taste profile.

TO MAKE THE CHICKEN

1. Preheat the oven to 350°F.

2. Place a large ovenproof skillet over medium–high heat and add the olive oil.

3. Brown the chicken on both sides, about 5 minutes total.

4. In a small bowl, whisk together the honey, mustard, paprika, and thyme.

5. Brush the honey mixture over the breasts and bake the chicken in the skillet until it is cooked through, about 25 minutes.

6. Serve with a generous scoop of the vegetable salsa.

TO MAKE THE SALSA

1. While the chicken is cooking, in a medium bowl, toss together the fennel, yellow beets, carrot, apple, lemon juice, and honey.

2. Season the slaw with sea salt and pepper.

3. Set aside.

ON THE SIDE: Parsnip-Celeriac Purée (page 81)

PREP TIP: The salsa can be made several days in advance and stored in the refrigerator in a sealed container. This allows the flavors to mellow and the vegetables to soften slightly.

Per Serving: Calories: 256; Fat: 7g; Protein: 25g; Total Carbs: 23g; Fiber: 4g; Sodium: 319mg

CHICKEN AND GINGER FRIED RICE

Gluten-Free • Dairy-Free • Nut-Free

SERVES 4

PREP: 10 minutes

COOK: 20 minutes

1 tablespoon olive oil

2 teaspoons sesame oil

½ sweet onion, chopped

2 teaspoons minced garlic

1 tablespoon grated fresh ginger

1 cup coarsely chopped baby bok choy

1 carrot, finely chopped

4 cups cooked brown basmati rice

2 cups chopped cooked chicken breast

2 tablespoons chopped fresh cilantro

2 tablespoons tamari

1 scallion, white and green parts, chopped

The most time-intensive part of making this simple dish is probably cleaning the baby bok choy. I am always surprised by the amount of dirt that can hide in the small creases of this vegetable, and have once made the mistake of not being thorough—nothing ruins a meal faster than gritty sauce! Rinse and scrub right down to the base of each baby bok choy before chopping them.

1. Place a large skillet over medium-high heat and add the olive oil and sesame oil.

2. Sauté the sweet onion, garlic, and ginger until softened, about 3 minutes.

3. Stir in the baby bok choy and carrots and sauté until softened, about 7 minutes more.

4. Add the rice, chicken, cilantro, and tamari.

5. Sauté, stirring constantly, for about 10 minutes, or until the rice and chicken are heated through.

6. Top with the scallion and serve.

ON THE SIDE: Pumpkin with Thyme (page 79)

VARIATION TIP: Fried rice is an extremely versatile dish that is delicious with almost any vegetable, meat, and even shrimp. Try beef, tofu, bean sprouts, and peppers in different combinations.

Per Serving: Calories: 300; Fat: 8g; Protein: 18g; Total Carbs: 40g; Fiber: 4g; Sodium: 557mg

CHICKEN-FETA BURGERS

Nut-Free • Kids Love It

SERVES 4

PREP: 15 minutes

COOK: 15 minutes

1 pound lean ground chicken

½ cup whole-wheat bread crumbs

2 celery stalks, finely chopped

1 small carrot, peeled and grated

1 scallion, white and green parts, chopped

½ cup crumbled low-sodium feta cheese

1 teaspoon minced garlic

2 teaspoons chopped fresh oregano

1 tablespoon olive oil

2 whole-wheat pitas, cut in half

1 tomato, chopped

2 tablespoons chopped black olives

The first time I served these chicken burgers to my family, I did not tell them what they had on their plates. The delight and appreciation of the cheesy herb-spiked patties inspired me to serve them every few weeks. If you need a gluten-free version, use ground almonds instead of bread crumbs and serve the burgers on a romaine-leaf "bun."

1. In a large bowl, combine the ground chicken, bread crumbs, celery, carrot, scallion, feta cheese, garlic, and oregano until well mixed.

2. Shape the chicken mixture into 4 equal-size patties.

3. Place a large skillet over medium-high heat and add the olive oil.

4. Pan sear the chicken burgers until cooked completely through, turning once, about 15 minutes.

5. Stuff the burgers into the pita-bread halves and top with the tomato and olives.

6. Serve.

ON THE SIDE: Avocado Chopped Salad (page 47)

VARIATION TIP: This recipe can also be made into tasty meatballs. Just roll the chicken mixture into balls using a tablespoon to measure the amount, and pan fry or bake them in the oven.

Per Serving: Calories: 358; Fat: 15g; Protein: 30g; Total Carbs: 27g; Fiber: 4g; Sodium: 506mg

MEDITERRANEAN CHICKEN THIGH BAKE

Gluten-Free • Dairy-Free • Nut-Free • Kids Love It

SERVES 4

PREP: 10 minutes

COOK: 40 minutes

1 tablespoon olive oil

4 (5-ounce) boneless chicken thighs

1 cup brown basmati rice

Sea salt

Freshly ground black pepper

2 cups sodium-free chicken broth

2 cups halved cherry tomatoes

1 red onion, sliced into eighths

½ cup pitted Kalamata olives

1 tablespoon chopped fresh basil

One-pot dinners save my sanity, because between two jobs, kids, dogs, cats, and regular life tasks I have no time to waste at dinnertime. This recipe leaves the skin on the chicken thighs to add flavor and moistness to the dish, but I usually remove it after the chicken is baked.

1. Preheat the oven to 375°F.

2. Place a large skillet over medium-high heat and add the olive oil.

3. Brown the chicken on both sides until golden, about 10 minutes total.

4. Spread the rice on the bottom of a 9-by-13-inch-deep baking dish.

5. Place the chicken on top.

6. Season the chicken with sea salt and pepper.

7. Add the chicken broth to the skillet and place it on high heat until it boils.

8. Scatter the cherry tomatoes, red onion, and olives between the chicken pieces and pour the boiling broth over everything.

9. Wrap the baking dish tightly with aluminum foil.

10. Bake until the chicken is cooked through, about 30 minutes.

11. Once cool enough to handle, remove the chicken skin (optional).

12. Top with the basil and serve.

PREP TIP: Assemble the entire recipe in advance and park it in the refrigerator until you get home for dinner. Bake for the same time and at the same temperature.

Per Serving: Calories: 378; Fat: 11g; Protein: 27g; Total Carbs: 43g; Fiber: 5g; Sodium: 235mg

FIERY CHICKEN-STUFFED EGGPLANT

Gluten-Free • Dairy-Free • Nut-Free

SERVES 4

PREP: 10 minutes

COOK: 35 minutes

2 small eggplants, cut in half lengthwise and the flesh scooped out leaving ½-inch shell

2 tablespoons olive oil, divided

1 pound lean ground chicken

½ sweet onion, chopped

2 teaspoons minced garlic

1 red bell pepper, chopped

1 sweet potato, chopped

2 cups chopped kale

1 (15-ounce) can sodium-free garbanzo beans

1 tomato, diced

2 tablespoons harissa

1 tablespoon chopped fresh basil

Due to its incredibly porous texture, eggplant soaks up fat and spices like a sponge. Eggplant is a common ingredient in Middle Eastern cooking, so using harissa to flavor this dish seemed like a natural choice. Harissa is a red hot-chili paste made with an assortment of ingredients including roasted red peppers and saffron. If you or anyone in your family has arthritis, consume eggplant and peppers in moderation because plants from the nightshade family can exacerbate symptoms.

1. Preheat the oven to 350°F.

2. Line a baking sheet with parchment paper.

3. Brush the eggplant halves with 2 teaspoons of olive oil and place them hollow-side up on the baking sheet.

4. While the eggplant is baking, place a large skillet over medium-high heat and add the remaining olive oil.

5. Sauté the ground chicken until it is heated through, about 5 minutes.

6. Stir in the sweet onion, garlic, red bell pepper, potato, and kale and sauté until the vegetables are softened, about 6 minutes.

7. Stir in the garbanzo beans, tomato, harissa, and basil.

8. Spoon the filling into the eggplant halves and bake until the eggplant is tender, about 15 to 20 minutes.

9. Serve.

ON THE SIDE: Baked Tomato Casserole (page 84)

PREP TIP: Use the scooped-out eggplant flesh for pasta sauce, soups, stews, and dips. This ingredient can be used to make a delicious baba ganoush if you have a favorite recipe.

Per Serving: Calories: 512; Fat: 18g; Protein: 34g; Total Carbs: 15g; Fiber: 16g; Sodium: 252mg

CREAMY CHICKEN CURRY

Gluten-Free • Nut-Free

SERVES 4

PREP: 5 minutes

COOK: 30 minutes

2 tablespoons olive oil

4 boneless, skinless chicken thighs

1 sweet onion, chopped

2 teaspoons minced garlic

1 teaspoon grated fresh ginger

1 (15-ounce) sodium-free diced tomatoes, undrained

½ cup coconut milk

2 tablespoons curry powder

½ cup plain yogurt

2 tablespoons chopped fresh cilantro

In North Africa there are many types of curries, but this tomato-based style is the most popular. The sauce is similar to tikka masala, and if you want to increase the similarity, use garam masala instead of plain curry powder in the same amount. Serve cucumber sticks with the curry to cut the heat of the spices.

1. In a large skillet over a medium-high heat, add the olive oil.

2. Pan sear the chicken thighs until they are browned all over, about 6 minutes.

3. Transfer the chicken to a plate and set aside.

4. Sauté the sweet onion, garlic, and ginger until they are softened, about 3 minutes.

5. Stir in the tomatoes, coconut milk, and curry powder.

6. Return the chicken to the skillet and bring the liquid to a boil.

7. Reduce the heat to low, cover the skillet, and simmer until the chicken is tender and the sauce is thick, about 20 minutes.

8. Serve topped with yogurt and cilantro.

ON THE SIDE: Brown basmati rice or quinoa

PREP TIP: Create your own curry seasoning using an assortment of traditional spices for the perfect combination. Cumin, coriander, turmeric, cinnamon, cardamom, ginger, clove, and black pepper can all be mixed in successfully.

Per Serving: Calories: 325; Fat: 19g; Protein: 26g; Total Carbs: 13g; Fiber: 4g; Sodium: 134mg

GOLDEN "FRIED" CHICKEN

· Kids Love It

SERVES 4

PREP: 10 minutes, plus 1 to 10 hours to marinate

COOK: 20 minutes

1½ cups unsweetened almond milk

½ cup plain yogurt

1 pound chicken drumsticks

2 cups whole-wheat bread crumbs

½ teaspoon smoked paprika

¼ teaspoon freshly ground black pepper

¼ teaspoon garlic powder

This dish has a color and satisfying crunch similar to that of fried chicken. You can use other parts of the chicken, but drumsticks are usually the most economical. I like to cut up a whole bird into wings, thighs, drumsticks, and breasts, but you have to adjust the cooking time to reflect the bigger pieces of poultry. If you go that route, remove smaller pieces as they are done and continue to cook until every piece registers a minimum of 165°F on a meat thermometer.

1. Whisk together the almond milk and yogurt until well blended.

2. Add the chicken to the almond-milk mixture, stirring to coat the pieces thoroughly.

3. Cover and marinate the chicken for 1 to 10 hours.

4. In a large bowl, stir together the bread crumbs, paprika, pepper, and garlic powder.

5. Preheat the oven to 450°F.

6. Line a baking sheet with foil and set aside.

7. Shake the excess liquid off the chicken and dredge each piece in the bread-crumb mixture to coat.

8. Place the chicken on the baking sheet and bake until the pieces are golden and crispy, about 20 minutes.

9. Serve.

ON THE SIDE: Succotash (page 76)

PREP TIP: Prepare the marinade and chicken in the morning before you go to work and let it sit until you are ready to make dinner. Bread the chicken and bake it while making whatever side dish you want to serve.

Per Serving: Calories: 325; Fat: 12g; Protein: 36g; Total Carbs: 15g; Fiber: 3g; Sodium: 272mg

SUN-DRIED TOMATO BRAISED CHICKEN

Gluten-Free • Dairy-Free • Nut-Free

SERVES 4

PREP: 5 minutes

COOK: 25 minutes

4 (4-ounce) boneless, skinless chicken breasts

Sea salt

Freshly ground black pepper

1 tablespoon olive oil

½ sweet onion, chopped

1 tablespoon minced garlic

1 (15-ounce) can sodium-free diced tomatoes, undrained

½ cup chopped sun-dried tomatoes

½ cup coconut milk

1 tablespoon chopped fresh basil

Sun-dried tomatoes are eaten as a snack in my house, so much so that I have to hide the jars if I want to use them in a specific recipe. Sun-dried tomatoes are a decent source of protein and fiber as well as potassium, iron, calcium, and vitamin K. This ingredient is packed with antioxidants that support heart health and boost immunity.

1. Preheat the oven to 375°F.

2. Lightly season the chicken breasts with sea salt and pepper.

3. Place a large ovenproof skillet over medium-high heat and add the olive oil.

4. Brown the chicken breasts on both sides, about 5 minutes total, and transfer to a plate.

5. Sauté the sweet onion and garlic until softened, about 3 minutes.

6. Stir in the tomatoes, sun-dried tomatoes, and coconut milk, and return the chicken breasts to the skillet.

7. Cover and place the skillet in the oven and braise until the chicken is tender, about 15 minutes.

8. Top with the basil and serve.

ON THE SIDE: Traditional Baked Beans with Collard Greens (page 86)

SUBSTITUTION TIP: Try making your own sun-dried tomatoes in the oven. Toss halved plum tomatoes with olive oil and bake in a 200°F oven for 8 hours. Store in the refrigerator for up to one week.

Per Serving: Calories: 360; Fat: 19g; Protein: 36g; Total Carbs: 12g; Fiber: 3g; Sodium: 288mg

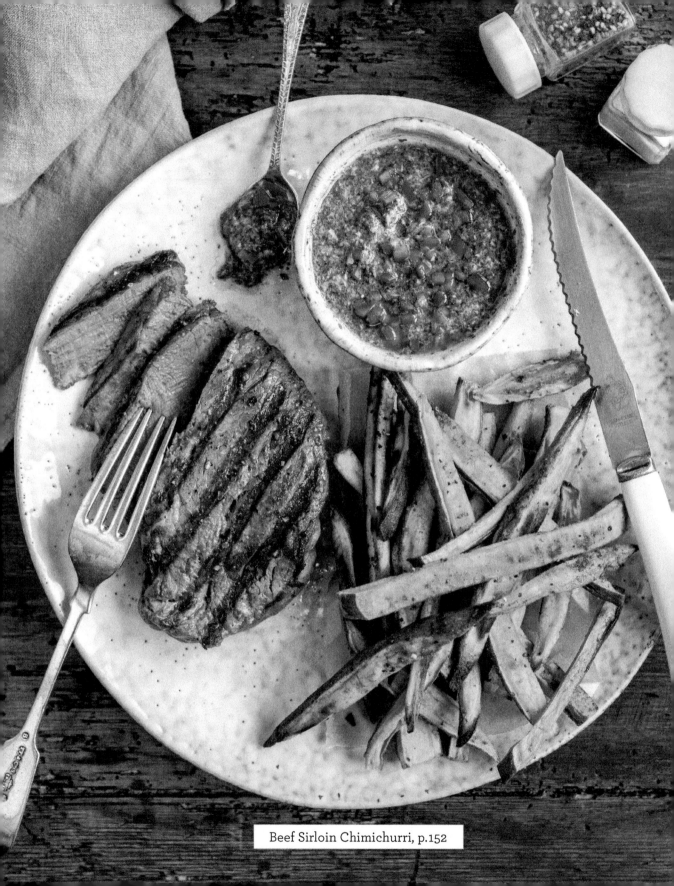

Beef Sirloin Chimichurri, p.152

10

MEAT

PORK LOIN WITH PEACH CHUTNEY

Gluten-Free • Dairy-Free • Nut-Free • Kids Love It

SERVES 4

PREP: 10 minutes

COOK: 20 minutes

FOR THE CHUTNEY

2 peaches, pitted and finely chopped

¼ cup unsweetened apple juice

¼ cup finely chopped sweet onion

1 tablespoon apple cider vinegar

1 tablespoon grated fresh ginger

2 teaspoons chopped fresh thyme

1 teaspoon fresh lemon zest

FOR THE PORK CHOPS

4 (5-ounce) pork chops

Sea salt

Freshly ground black pepper

1 tablespoon olive oil

In the Okanagan Valley, British Columbia, you can smell the peach orchards from several blocks away; the heady fragrance is intoxicating. Peach chutney tastes sweet, tart, and a little hot from the fresh ginger. Peaches are packed with nutrients such as fiber, beta carotene, vitamin C, and potassium. Including this juicy fruit in your diet regularly can help support weight loss and promote glowing skin.

TO MAKE THE CHUTNEY

1. In a small saucepan over medium heat, stir together the peaches, apple juice, sweet onion, vinegar, ginger, thyme, and lemon zest.

2. Cook, stirring occasionally, until the peaches become soft, about 10 minutes.

3. Remove the chutney from the heat and set aside.

TO MAKE THE PORK CHOPS

1. Preheat the oven to 400°F.

2. Season the pork chops with sea salt and pepper.

3. While the chutney is cooking, place a large ovenproof skillet over medium-high heat and add the olive oil.

4. Pan sear the pork on both sides until browned, about 5 minutes total.

5. Roast the pork chops in the oven until cooked through, about 10 minutes.

6. Serve with a generous spoonful of chutney.

ON THE SIDE: Golden Corn Pudding (page 83)

LEFTOVERS TIP: Store any leftover chutney in a sealed container in the refrigerator for up to four days. Try it as a spread on sandwiches or atop grilled chicken breast.

Per Serving: Calories: 320; Fat: 18g; Protein: 26g; Total Carbs: 10g; Fiber: 1g; Sodium: 234mg

PORK CHOPS WITH BLACK OLIVE TAPENADE

Gluten-Free • Dairy-Free • Nut-Free

SERVES 4

PREP: 10 minutes

COOK: 25 minutes

FOR THE TAPENADE

½ cup pitted Kalamata olives

3 tablespoons chopped fresh parsley

2 garlic cloves, peeled

2 tablespoons freshly squeezed lemon juice

1 tablespoon olive oil

FOR THE PORK CHOPS

4 (5-ounce) pork chops

Sea salt

Freshly ground black pepper

1 tablespoon olive oil

I remember the first time I made tapenade alongside a chef I greatly admired; the savory paste that we created for a rack of lamb delighted me. The tart, garlicky, rich creation works equally well with pork chops, and if you have some tapenade premade in the refrigerator, you can have dinner on the table in less than 30 minutes. Try green olives, different herbs, and even a pinch of red pepper flakes for unique variations on this tasty spread.

TO MAKE THE TAPENADE

1. Put the olives, parsley, garlic, lemon juice, and olive oil in a blender and pulse until the mixture is blended, but still slightly chunky.

2. Set aside.

TO MAKE THE PORK CHOPS

1. Preheat the oven to 400°F.

2. Season the pork chops with sea salt and pepper.

3. Place a large ovenproof skillet over medium-high heat and add the olive oil.

4. Pan sear the pork on both sides until browned, about 5 minutes total.

5. Spread the tapenade on the pork. Place the skillet in the oven and roast until just cooked through, about 15 minutes.

6. Serve.

ON THE SIDE: Parsnip-Celeriac Purée (page 81)

VARIATION TIP: Tapenade can be made with sun-dried tomatoes instead of olives—just use the same amount of the tomatoes. Store any leftover tapenade in the refrigerator in a sealed container for up to one week.

Per Serving: Calories: 334; Fat: 8g; Protein: 26g; Total Carbs: 2g; Fiber: 1g; Sodium: 378mg

BASIL-LAMB BURGERS

Nut-Free • Kids Love It

SERVES 4

PREP: 15 minutes

COOK: 10 minutes

1 pound ground lamb,
extra-lean

Sea salt

Freshly ground
black pepper

1 tablespoon olive oil

4 whole-grain
hamburger buns

¼ cup basil pesto

¼ cup low-sodium
feta cheese

1 tomato, cut into 8 slices

1 sweet onion, sliced thinly

1 cup chopped lettuce

Nothing says summer louder than the scent of burgers grilling on the barbecue on a balmy evening. These burgers are pan fried on the stove top but can be cooked on the grill as well. Lamb burgers can be any temperature—from rare to well-done—depending on your preference, so the timing will range from 8 minutes to about 15 minutes total.

1. Form the ground lamb into 4 equal patties and press them down to ½ inch thick.

2. Season the burgers on both sides with sea salt and pepper.

3. Place a large skillet on medium-high heat and add the olive oil.

4. Pan fry the lamb burgers until cooked to medium-well, turning once, about 10 minutes total.

5. Serve the lamb burgers on the buns with a tablespoon of pesto, feta cheese, sliced tomato, sweet onion, and lettuce.

ON THE SIDE: Roasted Summer Vegetables (page 75)

VARIATION TIP: Combining lamb, pork, and beef in the burgers can create a nice flavor and change the texture slightly. Choose extra-lean ground meats to keep the saturated fat content to an acceptable level.

Per Serving: Calories: 522; Fat: 25g; Protein: 29g; Total Carbs: 28g; Fiber: 7g; Sodium: 329mg

LAMB MEATBALLS IN CURRY SAUCE

Dairy-Free • Nut-Free • Kids Love It

SERVES 4

PREP: 10 minutes

COOK: 20 minutes

FOR THE MEATBALLS

1 pound ground lamb, extra-lean

1 carrot, grated, with the liquid squeezed out

¼ cup whole-wheat bread crumbs

1 scallion, white and green parts, chopped

1 teaspoon chopped fresh basil

1 teaspoon minced garlic

1 teaspoon grated fresh ginger

1 tablespoon olive oil

Meatballs are easy to prepare but do require a good mix of meat, fat, herbs, and sometimes fillers such as nut flour or bread crumbs. Too little fat or too much filler creates a dry and hard finished product. Lamb is a nice choice because this meat is naturally fatty and combines well with strong-flavored sauces or herbs. Throw together a double batch of the meatballs and freeze the cooked or raw extras for up to one month. Freeze them first individually on a baking tray before putting them in a bag, or you will end up with a solid mass rather than meatballs.

TO MAKE THE MEATBALLS

1. In a medium bowl, combine the ground lamb, carrot, bread crumbs, scallion, basil, garlic, and ginger until well mixed.

2. Roll the lamb mixture into meatballs, about 1 tablespoon per meatball.

3. Place a large skillet over medium-high heat and add the olive oil.

4. Brown the meatballs, turning a few times, about 5 minutes.

FOR THE SAUCE

1½ cups sodium-free chicken broth

½ cup coconut milk

1 tablespoon red curry paste

2 tablespoons sodium-free tomato paste

2 tablespoons chopped fresh cilantro

TO MAKE THE SAUCE

1. In a small bowl, whisk together the chicken broth, coconut milk, red curry paste, tomato paste, and cilantro.

2. Pour the sauce into the skillet with the meatballs and bring to a boil.

3. Reduce the heat to low and simmer until the meatballs are cooked through, about 15 minutes.

4. Serve.

ON THE SIDE: Brown basmati rice or couscous

LEFTOVERS TIP: Any leftover meatballs can be tucked cold into whole-wheat pita bread with a spoon of plain yogurt and some lettuce for a quick, filling lunch.

Per Serving: Calories: 398; Fat: 19g; Protein: 35g; Total Carbs: 12g; Fiber: 2g; Sodium: 260mg

BEEFY STUFFED TOMATOES

Nut-Free • Kids Love It

SERVES 4

PREP: 15 minutes

COOK: 20 minutes

Olive oil, for greasing
the baking dish

8 firm tomatoes, about
3 inches in diameter

1½ cups cooked,
extra-lean ground beef

1½ cups cooked
wheat berries

1 red bell pepper,
finely chopped

1 sweet onion,
finely chopped

2 tablespoons chopped
fresh parsley

2 teaspoons minced garlic

Freshly ground
black pepper

¼ cup goat cheese

Wheat berries might not be a familiar ingredient in your culinary repertoire, but you certainly have used whole-wheat flour, which is made from them. Once you try wheat berries, the slightly chewy texture and nutty taste will win you over. The convenience of this grain (it can be cooked and stored in the refrigerator for up to five days) is also a huge selling point. Wheat berries are a terrific source of fiber, B vitamins, and protein.

1. Preheat the oven to 375°F.

2. Lightly grease a shallow 9-by-13-inch baking dish and set aside.

3. Cut about ½ inch off the top of each tomato and carefully scoop out the pulp, leaving the shell. Arrange the tomato shells in the baking dish.

4. In a medium bowl, combine the beef, wheat berries, red bell pepper, sweet onion, parsley, and garlic. Season with pepper.

5. Spoon the filling into the tomatoes and crumble the goat cheese on top.

6. Bake the tomatoes until they are soft to the touch, about 15 to 20 minutes.

ON THE SIDE: Mixed green salad

VARIATION TIP: Bell peppers and zucchini make wonderful containers for filling instead of tomatoes. The peppers can be seeded to create a hollow, and the zucchini will need some of the flesh scooped out to create enough room.

Per Serving: Calories: 279; Fat: 7g; Protein: 26g; Total Carbs: 30g; Fiber: 7g; Sodium: 89mg

SUNDAY DINNER MEATLOAF

Nut-Free • Kids Love It

SERVES 4

PREP: 10 minutes

COOK: 45 minutes

1 pound extra-lean ground beef

½ cup whole-wheat bread crumbs

½ cup chopped sweet onion

½ cup grated carrots

1 teaspoon minced garlic

1 egg

2 tablespoons chopped fresh basil

1 teaspoon chopped fresh oregano

1 teaspoon chopped fresh parsley

Pinch sea salt

Pinch freshly ground black pepper

With two growing boys and a husband who works hard physically, meatloaf is an essential meal in my home because this dish does not cost very much to make and is very versatile. Any type of meat can be used along with a variety of vegetables, spices, and toppings. Meatloaf freezes beautifully, raw or cooked, so I always double up on my recipe and create an extra for a later date.

1. Preheat the oven to 350°F.

2. In a large bowl, combine the ground beef, bread crumbs, sweet onion, carrots, garlic, egg, basil, oregano, parsley, sea salt, and pepper until well mixed.

3. Press the meat mixture into a 9-by-5-inch loaf pan.

4. Bake the meatloaf until it is cooked through, about 45 minutes.

5. Let the meatloaf stand for 10 minutes, then tip out any accumulated grease.

6. Serve.

ON THE SIDE: Parsnip-Celeriac Purée (page 81)

LEFTOVERS TIP: Meatloaf sandwiches are a staple item on diner menus all over North America because they are comforting and delicious. Layer slices of cold meatloaf with whole-grain bread and enjoy.

Per Serving: Calories: 194; Fat: 5g; Protein: 26g; Total Carbs: 6g; Fiber: 1g; Sodium: 159mg

BEEF-BROCCOLI STIR-FRY

Gluten-Free • Dairy-Free • Kids Love It

SERVES 4

PREP: 10 minutes
COOK: 20 minutes

FOR THE SAUCE

1 cup sodium-free
beef broth

2 tablespoons tamari

2 tablespoons honey

2 tablespoons cornstarch

1 tablespoon minced garlic

2 teaspoons grated
fresh ginger

FOR THE STIR-FRY

1 tablespoon olive oil

1 teaspoon sesame oil

1 pound beef sirloin, cut
into 2-inch-long strips

2 cups broccoli florets

2 cups green beans,
trimmed

1 zucchini, cut in half
horizontally and sliced

1 garlic clove, sliced

Stir-frying is a speedy culinary technique that produces tender-crisp vegetables and melt-in-your-mouth meats. Broccoli and beef are a classic stir-fry combination found on many restaurant menus. This dish is usually quite spicy but this version tones down the heat for a more mellow presentation. If you enjoy a kick to your meals, add a pinch of red pepper flakes to the sauce until you are satisfied with the flavor.

TO MAKE THE SAUCE

1. In a small bowl, whisk together the beef broth, tamari, honey, cornstarch, garlic, and ginger.

2. Set aside.

TO MAKE THE STIR-FRY

1. Place a large skillet over medium-high heat and add the olive oil and sesame oil.

2. Sauté the beef until it is just cooked through, about 10 minutes, and transfer to a plate.

3. Add the broccoli, green beans, zucchini, and garlic to the skillet, and sauté until tender crisp, about 6 minutes.

4. Stir in the beef and toss to combine.

5. Move the veggies and beef over to the side of the skillet and pour in the sauce.

6. Stir the sauce until it thickens, about 4 minutes.

7. Toss the sauce with the beef stir-fry to coat.

8. Serve.

ON THE SIDE: Brown basmati rice

VARIATION TIP: The charm of stir fries is that any vegetable is delicious, so use whatever is in your refrigerator. Carrots, cauliflower, bok choy, bean sprouts, and baby corn all work with the sauce.

Per Serving: Calories: 416; Fat: 18g; Protein: 40g; Total Carbs: 25g; Fiber: 5g; Sodium: 462mg

ROOT VEGETABLE SHEPHERD'S PIE

Gluten-Free • Nut-Free

SERVES 4

PREP: 10 minutes

COOK: 20 minutes

1 sweet potato, peeled and diced

1 celeriac, peeled and diced

¼ cup plain yogurt

1 teaspoon olive oil

1 pound extra-lean ground beef

1 sweet onion, chopped

2 teaspoons minced garlic

1 cup chopped cauliflower

2 carrots, thinly sliced

1 (28-ounce) can sodium-free diced tomatoes, drained

1 cup peas

1 tablespoon fresh chopped oregano

Sea salt

Freshly ground black pepper

If you want to be technical, this is a cottage pie, not a shepherd's pie, because it is made with beef instead of lamb, although the names are often used synonymously with each other. If you sprinkle bread crumbs on the topping you then create what is called Cumberland pie. Whatever you call this dish, it is homey and the best comfort food for the cool fall and winter months.

1. Place the sweet potato and celeriac in a large saucepan and cover them with 2 inches of water.

2. Bring the water to a boil, and then reduce the heat to medium and simmer until the vegetables are soft, about 15 minutes.

3. Drain the vegetables, then add the yogurt and mash until fluffy and smooth.

4. Cover and set aside.

5. While the vegetables are boiling, place a large skillet over medium-high heat, pour in the olive oil, and add the ground beef.

6. Sauté the beef until it is cooked through, about 5 minutes.

7. Add the sweet onion, garlic, cauliflower, and carrots and sauté until tender crisp, about 5 minutes.

8. Stir in the tomatoes, peas, and oregano and simmer for 10 minutes.

9. Season the beef mixture with sea salt and pepper.

10. Serve the beef mixture topped with the mashed root vegetables.

ON THE SIDE: Mixed green salad

PREP TIP: If you have time to bake this dish, transfer the beef mixture to a 9-by-13-inch casserole dish and top evenly with the mashed vegetables. Bake at 375°F until the topping is lightly browned, about 25 minutes.

Per Serving: Calories: 357; Fat: 10g; Protein: 37g; Total Carbs: 32g; Fiber: 9g; Sodium: 248mg

BEEF SIRLOIN CHIMICHURRI

Gluten-Free • Dairy-Free • Nut-Free

SERVES 4

PREP: 10 minutes

COOK: 12 minutes

FOR THE SAUCE

¼ cup coarsely chopped parsley

3 tablespoons apple cider vinegar

2 tablespoons minced garlic

2 tablespoons fresh basil

1 teaspoon red pepper flakes

¼ cup olive oil

Sea salt

Freshly ground black pepper

Chopped red bell pepper, for garnish (optional)

FOR THE BEEF

2 (8-ounce) sirloin steaks

Sea salt

Freshly ground black pepper

Chimichurri is either green (*chimichurri verde*) or red (*chimichurri rojo*) and features parsley, garlic, vinegar, and olive oil. This uncooked sauce is a perfect accompaniment to grilled or broiled meats such as beef, pork, lamb, or chicken. If you want to create the red version, add chopped tomatoes or red bell peppers to the preparation.

TO MAKE THE SAUCE

1. Pulse the parsley, vinegar, garlic, basil, and red pepper flakes in a blender until smooth.

2. Transfer the mixture to a small bowl and stir in the olive oil.

3. Season with sea salt and pepper and garnish with the bell pepper (if desired). Set aside.

TO MAKE THE BEEF

1. Preheat the oven to broil.

2. Lightly season the steaks with sea salt and pepper.

3. Place the steaks on a baking sheet and broil until the desired doneness, about 6 minutes per side for medium.

4. Let the steak stand for 10 minutes before slicing it thinly across the grain.

5. Serve topped with chimichurri sauce.

ON THE SIDE: Golden Corn Pudding (page 83)

LEFTOVERS TIP: Chimichurri sauce is wonderful to have on hand to spoon into soups and stews. Double the recipe and store the sauce in a sealed container in the refrigerator for up to one week.

Per Serving: Calories: 329; Fat: 19g; Protein: 35g; Total Carbs: 2g; Fiber: 0g; Sodium: 97mg

PAN-SEARED BALSAMIC BEEF TENDERLOIN

Gluten-Free • Dairy-Free • Nut-Free

SERVES 4

PREP: 10 minutes

COOK: 17 minutes

1 teaspoon garlic powder

1 teaspoon onion powder

½ teaspoon ground coriander

⅛ teaspoon sea salt

⅛ teaspoon freshly ground black pepper

4 (4-ounce) beef tenderloin steaks

2 tablespoons Dijon mustard

2 tablespoons olive oil

2 tablespoons balsamic vinegar

1 tablespoon chopped fresh parsley

As the name implies, beef tenderloin is a tender cut of beef, but as with better cuts, it is not overly flavorful, so it needs seasoning to enhance the taste. Spices, Dijon mustard, and balsamic vinegar do the trick in this recipe. Select a high-quality balsamic vinegar for the best results.

1. Preheat the oven to 400°F.

2. In a small bowl, stir together the garlic powder, onion powder, coriander, sea salt, and pepper.

3. Coat the beef with the mustard and sprinkle the spice mixture all over both sides of the steaks.

4. Place a large ovenproof skillet over medium-high heat and add the olive oil.

5. Sear the beef on all sides, turning, about 7 minutes total.

6. Place the beef in the oven for an additional 5 minutes (for medium-rare) to 10 minutes (for medium).

7. Let the beef rest for 5 minutes before serving.

8. Drizzle with the balsamic vinegar and top with the parsley.

9. Serve.

ON THE SIDE: Baked Tomato Casserole (page 84)

PREP TIP: Always let your beef come to room temperature before searing or grilling it so that the internal temperature is accurate and warm. This is especially important if you like your meat rare.

Per Serving: Calories: 282; Fat: 14g; Protein: 35g; Total Carbs: 2g; Fiber: 0g; Sodium: 262mg

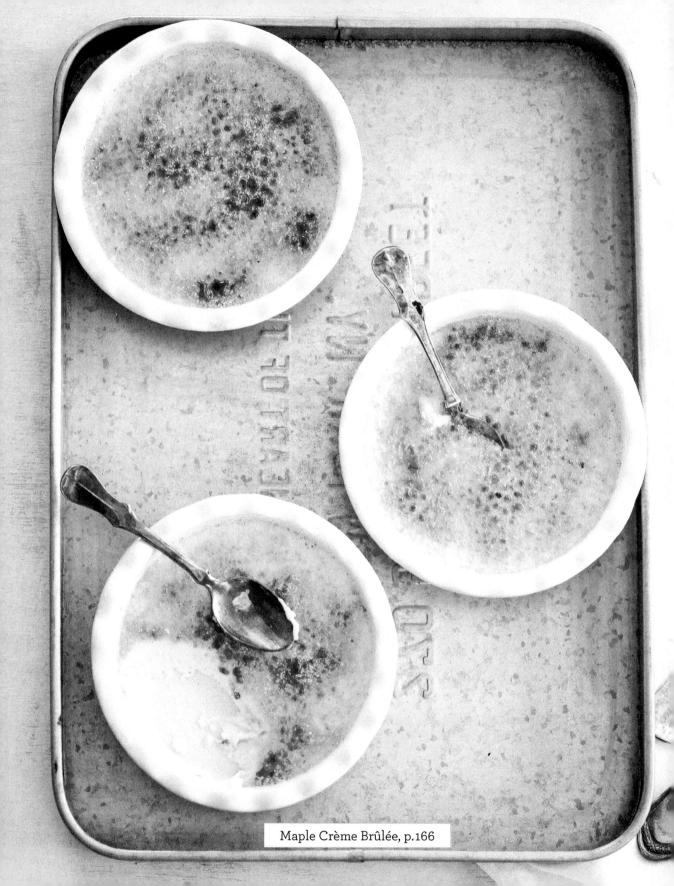

Maple Crème Brûlée, p.166

11

DESSERTS

GOAT CHEESE–STUFFED APPLES WITH PISTACHIOS

Gluten-Free • Vegetarian

SERVES 4

PREP: 10 minutes

COOK: 20 minutes

1 teaspoon melted coconut oil

2 apples, cored and hollowed out with a spoon

¼ teaspoon ground cinnamon

Pinch ground cloves

½ cup water

8 tablespoons (2 ounces) goat cheese

2 tablespoons maple syrup

¼ cup chopped pistachios

If you're a fan of cheesecake, this baked, lightly sweetened goat cheese tastes very similar. The apples you pick for the base should be a variety that is a little tart and firm, such as Cortland, Spartan, or McIntosh. Apples add lots of dietary fiber, especially from the skin, as well as small amounts of almost every other vitamin and mineral.

1. Preheat the oven to 350°F.

2. Place a medium skillet over medium heat and add the coconut oil.

3. Cut the apples in half. Sprinkle the cut sides of the apple halves with cinnamon and cloves, and place them skin-side up in the skillet.

4. Lightly brown them in the coconut oil, about 1 minute.

5. Place the apples in an 8-by-8-inch baking dish, hollow-side up, and pour in the water.

6. Roast the apples in the oven until softened, about 10 minutes, then remove from the oven.

7. In a small bowl, stir together the goat cheese and maple syrup.

8. Evenly divide the goat-cheese mixture between the apple halves, filling the hollows, and roast in the oven for 5 minutes.

9. Sprinkle the apples with pistachios and serve warm.

VARIATION TIP: You can use pears, peaches, or nectarines as the base of this simple scrumptious recipe. For the best results, pick ripe, firm fruit.

Per Serving (one apple half): Calories: 178; Fat: 8g; Protein: 5g; Total Carbs: 23g; Fiber: 3g; Sodium: 71mg

WHOLE-GRAIN FRUIT CRISP

Dairy-Free • Nut-Free • Vegan • Vegetarian • Kids Love It

SERVES 6

PREP: 10 minutes

COOK: 20 minutes

¼ cup coconut oil, melted, plus extra for greasing the baking dish

1 pear, peeled, cored, and cut into thin slices

1 cup raspberries

1 cup sliced strawberries

1 tablespoon maple syrup

½ teaspoon ground cinnamon

Pinch allspice

1 cup rolled oats

½ cup whole-grain flour

¼ cup maple sugar

Pinch sea salt

Apple crisp was the first dessert I learned to make from scratch, and it turned out so well that my father and sister picked off the entire golden crisp topping before dessert! This healthier whole-grain topping still has that tempting crunch and rich flavor. This dessert makes a special breakfast if there are any leftovers.

1. Preheat the oven to 375°F.

2. Lightly grease a 6-by-6-inch baking dish with coconut oil.

3. Mix together the pears, raspberries, strawberries, maple syrup, cinnamon, and allspice, and add the mixture to the baking dish.

4. In a small bowl, stir together the oats, flour, maple sugar, and sea salt.

5. Stir in the coconut oil and toss until the mixture resembles coarse crumbs.

6. Top the fruit evenly with the oat mixture.

7. Place the dish in the oven and bake until golden, about 20 minutes.

8. Serve warm.

VARIATION TIP: You can create delectable variations by changing the type of fruit used in the base of this dessert. Peaches, apples, blueberries, cherries, rhubarb, and blackberries should all be considered if ripe and seasonal.

Per Serving: Calories: 221; Fat: 9g; Protein: 4g; Total Carbs: 32g; Fiber: 4g; Sodium: 42mg

SWEET DESSERT OMELET

Gluten-Free • Dairy-Free • Nut-Free • Vegetarian • Kids Love It

SERVES 4

PREP: 10 minutes

COOK: 6 minutes

6 eggs

3 tablespoons maple syrup

2 tablespoons unsweetened shredded coconut

1 tablespoon ground flaxseed

½ teaspoon ground cinnamon

1 teaspoon coconut oil

1 banana, sliced

½ cup sliced strawberries

½ cup blueberries

I first sampled an *omelette au sucré* in Quebec, prepared at the table by the sous chef of the restaurant. It was like a soufflé without all the beating, folding, and careful baking. Basically, this dish was a bit of a revelation, so I went home and tried every filling I could think of under the sun, and with stellar results. Try this simple dessert for breakfast for a special occasion, as well.

1. In a medium bowl, whisk together the eggs, maple syrup, shredded coconut, flaxseed, and cinnamon until blended.

2. Place a large nonstick frying pan over medium-low heat and melt the coconut oil.

3. Pour in the egg mixture and cook, without disturbing, until the eggs are about three-quarters of the way cooked through and almost set, about 3 to 4 minutes.

4. Use a spatula to gently flip the omelet over and cook for 1 minute more.

5. Top with the banana, strawberries, and blueberries.

6. Fold the omelet over the filling and slide it onto a serving plate.

7. Cut into quarters and serve.

VARIATION TIP: Any fruit can be used to fill this simple, tempting dessert, so use whatever is ripe and seasonal in your area. Peaches, plums, cherries, apricots, oranges, and raspberries are all lovely choices.

Per Serving: Calories: 241; Fat: 10g; Protein: 10g; Total Carbs: 23g; Fiber: 3g; Sodium: 97mg

SWEET-POTATO PUDDING

Gluten-Free • Dairy-Free • Vegetarian • Kids Love It

SERVES 4

PREP: 5 minutes

COOK: 10 minutes

1½ cups unsweetened almond milk

1 cup puréed cooked sweet potatoes

3 eggs

¼ cup maple syrup

2 teaspoons pure vanilla extract

¼ cup arrowroot

1 teaspoon ground cinnamon

⅛ teaspoon ground nutmeg

Pinch sea salt

Pudding is a satisfying, homey dessert designed to wrap you up like a cozy blanket on a cold day. Sweet potatoes, a hint of maple syrup, and warm spices are the perfect blend for a delicious dessert. Don't worry if the pudding is a little lumpy when you start whisking everything together; the mashed sweet potatoes will smooth out as the dish heats up.

1. In a large saucepan over medium-high heat, whisk together the almond milk, sweet potatoes, eggs, maple syrup, vanilla, arrowroot, cinnamon, nutmeg, and sea salt.

2. Cook the pudding, whisking, until it thickens, about 10 minutes.

3. Remove the pudding from the heat and let it cool for about 10 minutes.

4. Serve warm, or refrigerate, covered, and serve cold.

PREP TIP: This pretty dessert is a good way to use up leftover baked sweet potatoes. Simply scoop the tender cooked potato out of the skins into a container and refrigerate until you want to make the pudding—it keeps for up to three days.

Per Serving: Calories: 228; Fat: 7g; Protein: 7g; Total Carbs: 32g; Fiber: 4g; Sodium: 169mg

ALMOND RICE PUDDING

Gluten-Free • Dairy-Free • Vegan • Vegetarian • Kids Love It

SERVES 4

PREP: 5 minutes

COOK: 20 minutes

1½ cups unsweetened almond milk

½ cup coconut milk

1 cup brown basmati rice

½ cup maple syrup

1 teaspoon pure vanilla extract

Pinch salt

Rice pudding might already be a common dish in your home, because this recipe is very old and easy. This version does not include the usual dairy products or sugar, which makes it much healthier for your family. The brown basmati adds a lovely nutty flavor and slightly chewy texture to the dessert. If you enjoy a creamier pudding, replace the rice with quinoa in the same amount.

1. In a medium saucepan over medium-high heat, add the almond milk, coconut milk, rice, maple syrup, vanilla, and salt.

2. Bring the rice mixture to a boil, and then reduce the heat to low and simmer until the rice is tender, stirring frequently, about 20 minutes.

3. Remove the pudding from the heat and serve warm.

LEFTOVERS TIP: Rice pudding is not only a fabulous dessert, it is also a satisfying breakfast if you want a treat. Top with fresh berries, sliced bananas, or chopped nuts.

Per Serving: Calories: 225; Fat: 7g; Protein: 2g; Total Carbs: 36g; Fiber: 3g; Sodium: 114mg

CHOCOLATE-ZUCCHINI BROWNIES

Gluten-Free • Dairy-Free • Vegetarian • Kids Love It

MAKES 8 BROWNIES

PREP: 10 minutes

COOK: 25 minutes

⅓ cup melted coconut oil, plus extra for greasing the baking dish

7 eggs

⅓ cup maple syrup

1 tablespoon pure vanilla extract

½ cup good-quality organic cocoa powder

½ cup coconut flour

1 teaspoon baking soda

¼ teaspoon sea salt

2 cups finely grated zucchini

The deep, dark-chocolate flavor of brownies is the perfect cover when you want to sneak some extra vegetables like zucchini into your family's diet. The bonus of this unexpected ingredient is the moistness it adds to this dessert. Look for quality cocoa from single-plantation suppliers or organic products for the richest taste and best health benefits.

1. Preheat the oven to 350°F.

2. Lightly grease an 8-by-8-inch baking dish with coconut oil and set aside.

3. In a large bowl, whisk together the eggs, coconut oil, maple syrup, and vanilla.

4. In a small bowl, stir together the cocoa powder, flour, baking soda, and salt.

5. Whisk the dry ingredients into the wet ingredients until well combined.

6. Stir in the zucchini until just mixed.

7. Bake the brownies for 25 minutes, until firm and a toothpick inserted in the center comes out clean.

8. Cool completely, cut into 8 squares, and serve.

VARIATION TIP: Brownies are delectable plain, but adding chopped pecans, walnuts, or hazelnuts adds a layer of crunch. Adding a few tablespoons of shredded, unsweetened coconut is also a wonderful choice if you crave a bit more texture.

Per Serving (1 brownie): Calories: 268; Fat: 15g; Protein: 9g; Total Carbs: 19g; Fiber: 6g; Sodium: 276mg

CHOCOLATE CUPCAKES

Vegetarian • Kids Love It

MAKES 12 CUPCAKES

PREP: 10 minutes

COOK: 30 minutes

1 cup almond flour

1 cup whole-wheat flour

½ cup good-quality cocoa powder

1½ teaspoons baking powder

½ teaspoon baking soda

Pinch sea salt

3 eggs

½ cup maple syrup

½ cup plain yogurt

¼ cup melted coconut oil

1 teaspoon pure vanilla extract

Who doesn't smile at the sight of cupcakes? Cupcakes are a culinary phenomenon with whole shops devoted to them, because people cannot get enough of these little gems. Coconut and chocolate is a scrumptious pairing, with just a hint of tartness from the yogurt. If you want a topping on these, try a little grated dark chocolate.

1. Preheat the oven to 350°F and line 12 muffin tins with paper liners. Set aside.

2. In a medium bowl, whisk together the almond flour, whole-wheat flour, cocoa powder, baking powder, baking soda, and sea salt until well combined.

3. In a large bowl, beat together the eggs, maple syrup, yogurt, coconut oil, and vanilla until combined, scraping down the sides of the bowl.

4. Add the dry ingredients to the wet ingredients and stir until just combined.

5. Spoon the batter into the prepared muffin tins.

6. Bake until a toothpick inserted in the center of the cupcakes comes out clean, about 30 minutes.

7. Remove the muffin tin from the oven and let the cupcakes cool on a wire rack for about 1 hour.

8. Store the cupcakes in a sealed container in the refrigerator for up to five days or wrap each cupcake individually and store in the freezer for up to two weeks.

VARIATION TIP: Dark-chocolate mini chips or chopped pecans can be stirred into the batter for texture and deeper flavor. Top them with whipped coconut cream as an extra treat.

Per Serving (1 cupcake): Calories: 161; Fat: 7g; Protein: 4g; Total Carbs: 21g; Fiber: 2g; Sodium: 98mg

MINT CHOCOLATE–CHIA MOUSSE

Gluten-Free • Dairy-Free • Vegan • Vegetarian • Kids Love It

SERVES 4

PREP: 15 minutes

COOK: 0 minutes

1½ cups unsweetened almond milk

5 tablespoons white chia seeds

2 tablespoons good-quality cocoa powder

2 tablespoons maple syrup

½ teaspoon pure mint extract

¼ cup coconut cream

Chocolate and chia are an exceptionally healthy fusion of ingredients because chocolate is packed with antioxidants—more than blueberries—and chia is an excellent source of fiber, protein, omega-3 fatty acids, and calcium. This is not as airy as a traditional mousse, but you can blitz the ingredients in a blender to create a smoother texture before letting it chill to thicken.

1. Stir together the almond milk, chia seeds, cocoa powder, maple syrup, and mint extract until very well blended.
2. Place the bowl in the refrigerator and chill, stirring every 5 minutes for the first 15 minutes.
3. Cover the mousse with plastic wrap and keep in the refrigerator until you wish to serve it.
4. In a medium bowl, whisk the coconut cream until it is fluffy and thick.
5. Top the mousse with the whipped cream and serve.

VARIATION TIP: You can leave out the mint extract if you want a plain chocolate dessert, or stir in mashed banana for a delectable flavor. Top with fresh berries and serve.

Per Serving: Calories: 192; Fat: 11g; Protein: 5g; Total Carbs: 20g; Fiber: 10g; Sodium: 76mg

TEMPTING ALMOND BUTTER CUPS

Gluten-Free • Dairy-Free • Vegetarian • Kids Love It

MAKES 12 CUPS

PREP: 15 minutes

COOK: 5 minutes

½ cup coconut oil

¼ cup good-quality cocoa powder

¼ cup maple syrup

¼ cup natural almond butter

2 tablespoons chopped almonds

Peanut-butter cups are the candy of choice for my family, including my father, who used to sort them out of my Halloween candy for his own enjoyment. These luscious almond cups taste quite similar to the peanut-butter originals and do not contain all the extra preservatives and sugar. They are an inspired choice when you want a little treat at the end of a large meal.

1. Line a 12-cup mini muffin tin with paper cups.

2. Place a small saucepan over medium-low heat and add the coconut oil, cocoa powder, maple syrup, and almond butter.

3. Stir until the mixture is melted and very smooth, about 5 minutes.

4. Spoon the mixture evenly between the cups and top with the chopped almonds.

5. Place the muffin tin in the refrigerator until the cups are firm.

6. Store the almond cups in a sealed container in the refrigerator for up to one week.

VARIATION TIP: Any nut butter works in the cups such as peanut butter, cashew butter, and pecan butter. Change the topping to reflect the type of nut butter in the base mixture.

Per Serving (1 cup): Calories: 167; Fat: 14g; Protein: 3g; Total Carbs: 8g; Fiber: 2g; Sodium: 23mg

MAPLE CRÈME BRÛLÉE

Gluten-Free • Dairy-Free • Vegetarian • Kids Love It

SERVES 4

PREP: 10 minutes

COOK: 50 minutes

1¾ cups unsweetened almond milk

5 egg yolks

¼ cup maple syrup

1 teaspoon pure vanilla extract

4 teaspoons maple sugar (optional)

Real maple syrup is an expensive product, but the cost is well worth it for the flavor and quality. If your syrup seems like a really good deal, check the label to rule out additives such as corn syrup. The best grade to use for this recipe is dark with a rich caramel taste, Grade B Dark Amber.

1. Preheat the oven to 300°F.

2. Place 4 (4-ounce) ramekins in a small baking dish and pour enough water into the dish to come about halfway up the sides of the ramekins.

3. Place the almond milk in a medium saucepan over medium-low heat, and heat until it just begins to steam, about 4 minutes. Remove from the heat.

4. In a medium bowl, whisk together the egg yolks, maple syrup, and vanilla.

5. Whisk in the almond milk and pour the mixture through a fine-mesh sieve into the ramekins.

6. Place the baking dish in the oven and bake until set, about 45 minutes.

7. Remove the baking dish from the oven and transfer the ramekins to a wire rack.

8. Cool completely and chill in the refrigerator.

9. If you want a true crème brûlée, sprinkle the tops with maple sugar and broil the brûlée in the oven until the sugar is caramelized.

10. Serve.

SUBSTITUTION TIP: Skim milk and coconut milk can be used instead of almond milk. You can also add chopped mango, raspberries, and blueberries to create delectable pockets of sweetness in the dessert.

Per Serving: Calories: 137; Fat: 7g; Protein: 4g; Total Carbs: 15g; Fiber: 1g; Sodium: 91mg

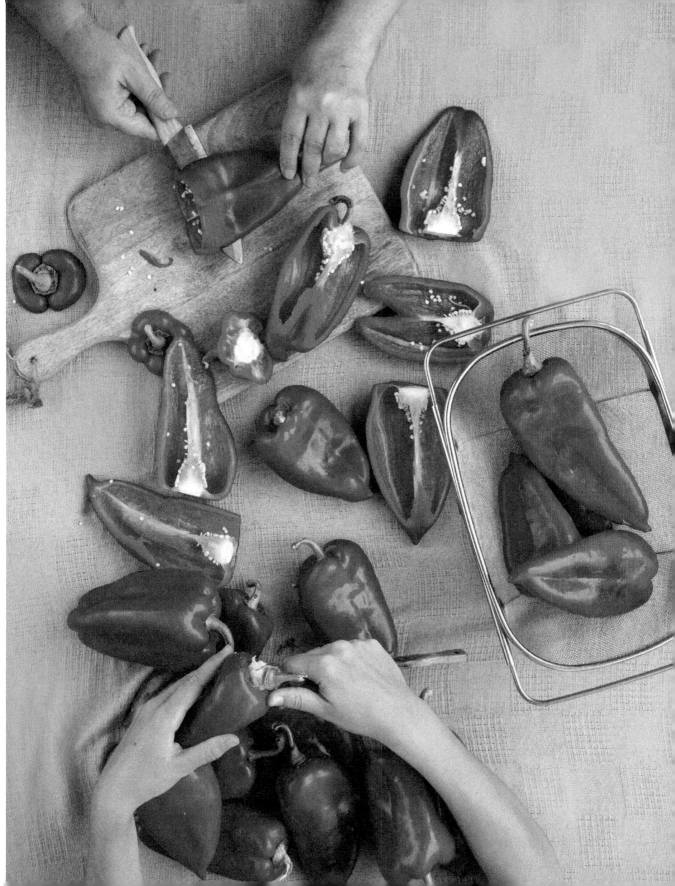

THE DIRTY DOZEN AND CLEAN FIFTEEN

A nonprofit environmental watchdog organization called Environmental Working Group (EWG) looks at data supplied by the US Department of Agriculture (USDA) and the Food and Drug Administration (FDA) about pesticide residues. Each year it compiles a list of the best and worst pesticide loads found in commercial crops. You can use these lists to decide which fruits and vegetables to buy organic to minimize your exposure to pesticides and which produce is considered safe enough to buy conventionally. This does not mean they are pesticide-free, though, so wash these fruits and vegetables thoroughly.

These lists change every year, so make sure you look up the most recent one before you fill your shopping cart. You'll find the most recent lists, as well as a guide to pesticides in produce, at EWG.org/FoodNews.

DIRTY DOZEN

Apples
Celery
Cherries
Cherry tomatoes
Cucumbers
Grapes
Nectarines
Peaches
Spinach
Strawberries
Sweet bell peppers
Tomatoes

In addition to the Dirty Dozen, the EWG added two types of produce contaminated with highly toxic organophosphate insecticides:

Kale/Collard greens
Hot peppers

CLEAN FIFTEEN

Asparagus
Avocados
Cabbage
Cantaloupe
Cauliflower
Eggplant
Grapefruit
Honeydew melon

Kiwifruits
Mangos
Onions
Papayas
Pineapples
Sweet corn
Sweet peas (frozen)

MEASUREMENT CONVERSIONS

VOLUME EQUIVALENTS (LIQUID)

US STANDARD	US STANDARD (OUNCES)	METRIC (APPROXIMATE)
2 tablespoons	1 fl. oz.	30 mL
¼ cup	2 fl. oz.	60 mL
½ cup	4 fl. oz.	120 mL
1 cup	8 fl. oz.	240 mL
1½ cups	12 fl. oz.	355 mL
2 cups or 1 pint	16 fl. oz.	475 mL
4 cups or 1 quart	32 fl. oz.	1 L
1 gallon	128 fl. oz.	4 L

OVEN TEMPERATURES

FAHRENHEIT	CELSIUS (APPROXIMATE)
250°F	120°C
300°F	150°C
325°F	165°C
350°F	180°C
375°F	190°C
400°F	200°C
425°F	220°C
450°F	230°C

VOLUME EQUIVALENTS (DRY)

US STANDARD	METRIC (APPROXIMATE)
⅛ teaspoon	0.5 mL
¼ teaspoon	1 mL
½ teaspoon	2 mL
¾ teaspoon	4 mL
1 teaspoon	5 mL
1 tablespoon	15 mL
¼ cup	59 mL
⅓ cup	79 mL
½ cup	118 mL
⅔ cup	156 mL
¾ cup	177 mL
1 cup	235 mL
2 cups or 1 pint	475 mL
3 cups	700 mL
4 cups or 1 quart	1 L

WEIGHT EQUIVALENTS

US STANDARD	METRIC (APPROXIMATE)
½ ounce	15 g
1 ounce	30 g
2 ounces	60 g
4 ounces	115 g
8 ounces	225 g
12 ounces	340 g
16 ounces or 1 pound	455 g

RECIPE INDEX

INDEX

ABOUT THE AUTHOR

MICHELLE ANDERSON is a mother and professional chef. Inspired by her own mother's green thumb as a child, Michelle has dedicated her career to promoting the benefits of a toxin-free lifestyle, making it easy to say goodbye to processed foods with her wholesome recipes. She is the author of *The No-Fuss Bread Machine Cookbook* and *Salads That Inspire*.

CPSIA information can be obtained
at www.ICGtesting.com
Printed in the USA
BVOW11s0520170817
492300BV00004B/9/P